Health Essentials

Colour Therapy

Pauline Wills runs a thriving practice in Reflexology and
Colour Therapy in London. She also works with the Hygeia
College of Colour Therapy and gives talks and workshops
throughout Europe.

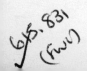

The Health Essentials Series

There is a growing number of people who find themselves attracted to holistic or alternative therapies and natural approaches to maintaining optimum health and vitality. The *Health Essentials* series is designed to help the newcomer by presenting high quality introductions to all the main complementary health subjects. Each book presents all the essential information on a particular therapy, explaining what it is, how it works and what it can do for the reader. Advice is also given, where possible, on how to begin using the therapy at home, together with comprehensive lists of courses and classes available worldwide.

The *Health Essentials* titles are all written by practising experts in their fields. Exceptionally clear and concise, each text is supported by attractive illustrations.

Series Medical Consultant
Dr John Cosh MD, FRCP

In the same series

Acupuncture by Peter Mole
Alexander Technique, by Richard Brennan
Aromatherapy by Christine Wildwood
Ayurveda by Scott Gerson MD
Chi Kung by James MacRitchie
Chinese Medicine by Tom Williams PhD
Flower Remedies by Christine Wildwood
Herbal Medicine by Vicki Pitman
Homeopathy by Peter Adams
Iridology by James & Sheelagh Colton
Kinesiology by Ann Holdway
Massage by Stewart Mitchell
Natural Beauty by Sidra Shaukat
Reflexology by Inge Dougans with Suzanne Ellis
Self-Hypnosis by Elaine Sheehan
Shiatsu by Elaine Liechti
Spiritual Healing by Jack Angelo
Vitamin Guide by Hasnain Walji

Health Essentials

COLOUR THERAPY

the use of colour
for health and healing

PAULINE WILLS

E L E M E N T
Shaftesbury, Dorset ● Rockport, Massachusetts
Brisbane, Queensland

© Element Books Limited 1993
Text © Pauline Wills 1993

First published in Great Britain in 1993 by
Element Books Limited
Shaftesbury, Dorset SP7 8BP

Published in the USA in 1993 by
Element Books, Inc.
42 Broadway, Rockport, MA 01966

Published in Australia in 1993 by
Element Books Limited
for Jacaranda Wiley Limited
33 Park Road, Milton, Brisbane 4064

Reprinted 1994
Reprinted 1995
Reprinted 1996

This edition 1997

Cover design and illustration by Max Fairbrother
Design by Nancy Lawrence
Illustrations by Taurus Graphics & David Gifford
Typeset by The Electronic Book Factory, Fife
Printed and bound in Great Britain by
Biddles Limited, Guildford & King's Lynn

British Library Cataloguing in Publication
data available

Library of Congress Cataloging in Publication
data available

ISBN 1–86204–044–3

Note from the Publisher

Any information given in any book in the *Health Essentials* series is not intended to be taken as a replacement for medical advice. Any person with a condition requiring medical attention should consult a qualified medical practitioner or suitable therapist.

Contents

Introduction

WHEREVER YOU MAY be reading this book, stop for a moment and look around you. What does your attention focus on? Is it furnishings, objects, people – or the colours pertaining to these things? Look again, but this time pay attention to the colours.

If you are in your own home, ask yourself why you chose the colour scheme which is displayed in your decorations and furnishings. Was it because they happened to be your favourite colours or was it because they have a psychological effect upon you – because they make you feel 'good', happy or relaxed?

The same question applies to the clothes you are wearing. Did you put them on because they were the nearest thing to hand, or did you wear them because of their colour?

These may be questions which you have never thought to ask yourself. If this is so, allow yourself a short space of time to reflect on them.

We are constantly surrounded by colour, which most people take for granted. Those who work with colour, however, such as artists, designers and colour therapists, become acutely sensitive to its physical and psychological effects.

The colours displayed in nature are awe inspiring. If you carefully examine the petals of a red rose, you will discover that each one has its own hue and variations of colour which can range from the deepest red to the palest shade of pink.

When its buds start to open, a tree reveals pale green leaves which darken as spring turns to summer, and which change again into orange, gold, yellow and brown, as autumn arrives.

1

Birds too are noted for their beautiful colours, particularly in the exotically coloured plumage of the male bird in courtship. Think of the peacock with its wonderful tail, or the parrot with its myriad multi-coloured feathers.

We can also perceive colour through the eyes of artists, each one bringing before us his or her own interpretation of colour and how it can be used. Normal everyday scenes can be transformed into vibrant or serene masterpieces when placed in the hands of an outstanding artist. For example, the paintings of Pièrre Bonnard seem to radiate a love and understanding of colour which penetrates and floods our senses.

Colour perceived as a surface colour, whether in nature or elsewhere, is known as a pigment colour. To our ancestors, the chemistry of colour was akin to that of alchemy. As certain colours could only be produced from rare materials it was only the wealthy or élite who were able to have them. Not possessing our understanding of science and technology which enables us to produce colours synthetically, the colour dyes which our ancestors produced were 'natural', made by extracting colours from nature.

The way in which we use our abundance of colour choice today is, to some extent, influenced by past generations. The breathtaking works of ancient Egypt are lasting evidence of the source to which most Western art and architecture can be traced. The Egyptians took their inspiration from their surroundings – the intensity of the desert sun and the fertility of the Nile Valley.

The Romans delighted in brilliantly coloured murals and mosaics, and a love of vibrant colour is also very apparent in Islamic art, particularly in their calligraphy and stylized floral designs.

Africa, too, seems wreathed in magic and filled with subtle colour. Those African tribes who lead a very simple life and have a strong bond with nature, display the colours of the earth in their homes. Their homes are made of mud and clay, but the interior walls are at times polished to such a high gloss that they act like mirrors, reflecting the light. The people's clothes and the interiors of their homes frequently display blue, white and green. More vivid colour, however, which they believe to contain a more powerful vibration and influence, is reserved for ritual decoration – the painting of their bodies in times of

2

war and festivity, the decoration on the face masks worn for fertility and initiation rites, and the richness of design in the amulets which adorn their bodies.

The country where colour seems to be most alive is India, possibly a reflection of the bright, hot climate. This vitality can be seen in the vivid, sometimes gaudy, colours of the saris worn by Indian women, it is also present in their art and craft work. Colours play an important part in Hindu worship, specific colours being ascribed to many of their gods. Vermilion and ochre, for example, represent blood in sacrificial rites; brides are sprinkled with turmeric; and yellow clothes are worn, and yellow food eaten, at the Spring Festival to symbolize the ripening of the crops. Bright pigments are sold to worshippers to enable them to paint their faces before taking part in religious ceremonies. At the festival of *Holi*, the celebration of Krishna's visit to earth, people throw coloured powder and water over each other.

The American Indians lived in perfect harmony with nature, and we can see evidence of this reflected in the patterns and colours depicted in their crafts. These symbolized the elements of their surroundings: the reds and browns of the earth; the blues and indigo of the sky; the white of the water; and the green of foliage. They calculated time by the amount of light radiating from the sun, and they knew the seasons of the year from the changing colours of the trees. Their decorative skills, displayed in their clothing, beadwork, quill-stitching, and body-painting, also contained a mystical presence. For example, they decorated both the outside and the inside of their *tipis* with representational pictures of their dreams and the battles they had won. When they moved – a frequent occurrence – and sold their *tipi*, they also sold the magic and the good fortune which the drawings were thought to procure.

From these examples, and others such as the richly extrovert colour heritage of Latin America, we can learn that colour has always played a vital role in many cultures and religions throughout the world.

The most beautiful phenomenon of colour is the rainbow. This arc of colour is caused by refraction and internal reflection of light in raindrops, causing the breaking up of the white light into the eight colours of the spectrum, in varying degrees of intensity according to the size of the raindrops. The colours which appear are red, orange, yellow, green, turquoise, blue, violet and magenta. Sometimes, in brilliant sunshine, a second or even a third bow, in fainter colours, may be seen. This spectacle is classified as colour illumination. The difference between colour illumination and colour pigment lies in the fact that pigments reflect a colour, transmitting the colours they cannot absorb. Colour illumination, however, saturates the space being illuminated with colour.

Another beautiful and awe-inspiring colour spectacle is the great display of polar lights, known as the aurora borealis. Scientists describe these as large effulgent magnetic fields. R. A. Madhill, a Canadian astronomer, who has carried out extensive research into this phenomenon, believes that the aurora borealis is caused by an invisible energy from the sun and is allied to the earth's magnetism. He came to these conclusions because the area where the lights are most frequently seen is near the earth's north magnetic pole. He also discovered that in the area where these lights are displayed to their maximum, there occur both magnetic and electric disturbances. People who have been in the midst of these lights talk about receiving an energizing force which fades with the fading of the lights.

If we penetrate into the heart of mountains, into caves and beneath the crust of the earth, we will find crystals growing in the darkness. When brought out into the open, these reveal a beautiful spectrum of coloured light. However solid a crystal may appear, it contains life force which makes it into a living structure. The growth and formation of a crystal is a continuous process, and it is virtually impossible to specify the length of time that a crystal takes to form.

During its growth process in the darkness of the earth, each crystal follows a precise geometric form, such as that of a cube, octahedron or tetrahedron. And, depending on the composition of minerals which go into its formation, each type of crystal will display a different colour. For example:

Red   – ruby and garnet
Orange   – carnelian and orange jasper
Yellow   – amber and yellow topaz
Green   – emerald and malachite

Blue   – sapphire and lapiz lazuli
Violet   – amethyst and fluorite
Magenta   – rose quartz

For centuries crystals have been used in healing all over the world. In India, for example, there is a form of gem therapy closely aligned to ayurvedic medicine. Ayurvedic medicine is often referred to as the science of life and has its roots in India. It treats the whole person, that is, the mental, emotional, spiritual and physical aspects and not just the symptoms. According to Ayurveda, health is the state of balance of the three doshas which are *vata* (wind), relating to the elements of air and ether; *pitta* (bile) relating to the elements of fire and earth and *kapha* (phlegm) relating to the elements of ether and water. An ayurvedic practitioner's concern is to determine which dosha has been vitiated and to treat accordingly. Treatment consists of a strict diet regime and the taking of prescribed ayurvedic medicine.

Indian gem therapists believe that everything is composed of the seven rays which are primeval, formative forces of nature, and it is through the combination of these forces that tangible forms are produced. Therefore, if a person is suffering some form of disease, they need to be treated with the appropriate colour or colours. This is done using gem stones, for gem therapists believe that these are the storehouse of cosmic colour. There are several methods of extracting the colour from the stones. One is to burn them to ash which is then administered to the patient. Another method is to store the stones in alcohol for seven days, allowing the vibrations of the colour to be absorbed into the alcohol. This is then given to the patient in homoeopathic proportions. The third method, which is primarily used for absent healing, is to put the gems on to a silver disc. This is then rotated at 1,400 rpm in front of a photograph of the person who has requested treatment.

I learnt about these techniques from an Indian patient who had been treated by gem therapy in India. He had suffered for many years with digestive problems and these had become so acute that he was only able to drink milk or water. Conventional medicine had been unable to diagnose the problem or alleviate the symptoms so he returned to India and was treated for six months with this method. He told me that he benefited greatly from it, that the symptoms subsided, and he was once again able to take solid food.

I first became interested in colour therapy through my study and practice of yoga. Through studying yoga philosophy I learnt about the subtle anatomy of a human person (see Chapter 3). The subtle anatomy is a cascade of continuously changing colours, embracing all the shades contained in each colour of the spectrum. I longed to know more.

Quite by chance, a girlfriend saw a course on 'colour therapy' advertised in her local library. I telephoned the number given, and enrolled for the course, after which I spent some time each week at the school, under the guidance of the principals, working with sick people. At this time there was very little public awareness about colour therapy. This usually meant that the people who came for treatment were nearly always terminally ill, and they looked upon this treatment as their last hope. Through treating these people with colour, under excellent supervision, I experienced some amazing results. Not everyone was restored to health, but pain was relieved in those who were dying and they became more relaxed and able to talk about death. From the experience that I was gaining, and the results which I was seeing, I knew that colour was a very powerful force, and I wanted to learn more about it.

Several years later, whilst attending a health exhibition, I met the principal of another school of colour healing. His approach and methods were different, but I knew that I could learn a great deal from the two-year course he was running. I found it absorbing and exciting. When I had completed the course, and started to run my own practice of colour therapy, I integrated the teachings from both schools, taking from each what I felt was right for me.

This was the foundation upon which I stood and started to grow.

I have now been working with, and teaching, colour therapy for many years, and it still holds wonder and amazement for me. It works with the 'whole' person – body, mind and spirit – and during treatment I find that old barriers are broken down and blockages released, allowing the energy to flow again freely, healing any existing dis-ease.

In colour therapy, as in all complementary therapies, the patient must work with the practitioner. Through allopathic medicine, many people have been conditioned to believe that all they have to do in order to become well is to take certain drugs at set intervals throughout the day. This is not the case with complementary therapies. Here, the human body is likened to a beautiful piece of machinery which, given the right conditions, is self-repairing. If it becomes ill, then there is a cause, which may be physical, emotional, metabolic or mental. Once the cause is eradicated, the ailment will start to heal itself. This seems simple in theory, but can be very difficult in practice, for there are times when a person knows the cause, but is unable to do anything about it. Similarly, the person may have buried the cause in their unconscious mind because they have found it too painful to cope with. This is where counselling plays a major part. There are many people in the world who are either extremely lonely or who have nobody close enough to trust or confide in. The therapist frequently fills this space and, in order to do this, we have to learn to be good listeners.

Having said this, I feel it important to stress that complementary therapies should complement and not replace orthodox medicine. The ideal situation is one in which a doctor and therapist work side by side, each respecting and acknowledging the other's work. When a patient comes to see me for the first time, I ask them if they have been to see their own doctor. If not, I always recommend that they do so. If they choose not to take this advice, then the responsibility is theirs. Like many of my colleagues, I am not a qualified doctor, and am not in a position to make a medical diagnosis.

Many people may look at the title of this book, *Colour Therapy*, or may glance through the first few pages, before putting it back on the shelf in disbelief. I too might have done this at an earlier stage in my life. All I can ask is that you do not dismiss it before you have examined it more closely. I know that it works but you do not have take my word for it – go and prove it for yourself.

I would like to end this introduction with the case history of a patient whom I shall call Mrs X.

Mrs X came for advice after discovering a lump in her right breast. She was asked if she had consulted her own GP and she said that she had. He had examined her and confirmed her findings. A hospital appointment was arranged so that the lump could be aspirated for the purpose of a biopsy. Mrs X stressed that she did not want this done. She believed that if the lump was malignant, any interference with it could spread the malignant cells.

After a lengthy discussion about her decision, colour treatment was started. After each treatment, she was given colour visualization and affirmation exercises to carry out two to three times a day. She was also advised on her diet and her level of stress.

At the end of three months, she reported that the lump appeared to be smaller. This gave her great hope and determination to carry on with the treatment. This continued for a further three months, during which time the lump became smaller and smaller until it finally disappeared. Mrs X was delighted and is now a great believer in colour therapy.

In *Body the Shrine, Yoga the Light* by B. K. S. Iyenger, the question is asked 'Who is a truly healthy man?' This is the answer given:

A person who has his physical, mental and spiritual personalities well under control and is trying to integrate the energies of his body and mind to fuse with the total energy of the universe – he is a man people can approach with their troubles – mental, physical and spiritual. Such were the rishis of old, living in the absolute present without any regrets for their past nor any anxieties for the future.

What wonderful food for thought.

1

What is Colour Therapy?

TO ANSWER THIS question very simply, colour therapy involves treating a person with colour rays in order to bring their body back into harmony, thereby restoring health and well-being. The application of colour can be rendered in many ways, which will be described in a later chapter.

From reading the introduction you will have learned that colour plays a very important role in our lives. We are constantly surrounded by it in its many manifestations. It has the power to evoke inner feelings and memories, and possesses a language of its own. How many times have we heard or used the expressions: 'green with envy', 'a black mood', 'red with anger', 'feeling blue', and 'white as a sheet'? Used as an energy, colour has the power to calm, excite, inspire, balance, manipulate, bring about a state of harmony, and to heal. It works on all three levels of our being – body, mind and spirit.

Colour is derived from light. In the beginning was the sacred darkness, and God said: 'Let there be light.' From this darkness the light poured forth, and the light gave birth to the colours of the spectrum.

One way of experiencing this phenomenon, is to shine light through a prism. The prism refracts the light and splits it up into the eight colours of red, orange, yellow, green, turquoise, blue, violet and magenta (see Fig. 1).

Now place the prism on to the bridge of your nose and look through it at the objects around you. You should discover that each object is surrounded by these beautiful colours.

9

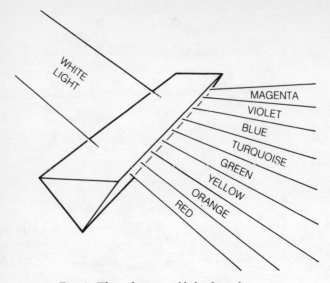

Fig. 1. The refraction of light through a prism

THE ELECTROMAGNETIC SPECTRUM

Colour is a form of radiation, and forms part of the electromagnetic spectrum. The electromagnetic spectrum starts with radio waves, which have a low frequency and long wave lengths, and rises through infra-red rays, visible light, ultraviolet light, x-rays, gamma rays, and cosmic rays. As we work through this spectrum, the wave lengths become shorter and the frequency higher, cosmic rays possessing the shortest wave lengths and the highest frequency. With the obvious exception of the visible rays, all of these are invisible to human sight and, apart from the cosmic rays about which very little is known, these invisible rays are used in science and medicine – sometimes with horrendous side effects. The visible light which falls in the middle of this spectrum contains the eight colours of the spectrum. It is not the case that because we are able to see them, they have no effect on us; like all the other rays, they are a form of radiation and can affect us in very subtle ways.

The wave lengths of visible light are the same as those of the sun when it reaches the earth at its greatest strength. These wave lengths lie approximately between 400 and 700

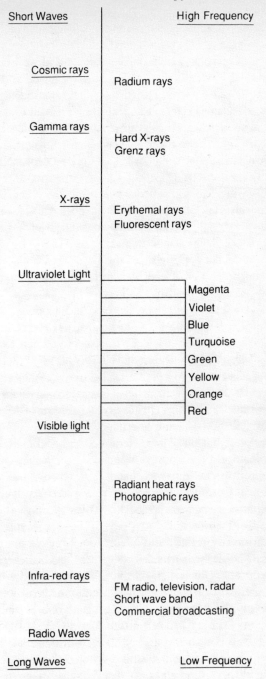

Fig. 2. The Electromagnetic Spectrum

nanometers, a nanometer being equivalent to one billionth of a metre.

We are creatures which derive our life and well-being from the sun. We have all experienced how depressed and lethargic we can become in winter with its short days and lack of sun. This is sometimes referred to as the 'winter blues'.

It has been reported in countries such as Finland, Sweden and Norway, where there is very little sunlight during the winter months, that the people succumb to depression, illness and lethargy, often resorting to alcohol and drugs. Albert Szert-Gyorki, the author of an article on 'Bioelectronics', and K. Martinek and I. V. Berezin, co-authors of an article on 'Artificial Light-Sensitive Enzymatic Systems as Chemical Amplifiers of Weak Light Signals', have carried out research into the effects of sunlight on the body, and have found that it affects the power of enzymes and hormones, often causing dynamic reactions within the body.

The Ancient Egyptians, Greeks and Romans were well known for using sunlight to aid healing. The Greek historian Herodotus (484–424 BC) is reputed to have been the founder of this form of healing, known as 'heliotherapy'. Heliotherapy was first used on a large scale by Bernard (1902) and Rollier (1903), in Switzerland, where it was chiefly employed in sanatoriums for the prevention and treatment of tuberculosis. One of the active components of the sun's emanations is ultraviolet radiation. Heliotherapy is also beneficial in cases of eczema and other skin problems.

A condition which was first identified and named by Dr Norman E. Rosenthal in 1981, is Seasonal Affective Disorder, more commonly known as 'SAD'. This condition starts at the beginning of winter and disappears in the spring. It is caused by deprivation of sunlight and affects four times as many women as men. People with this disorder suffer severe depression and increased appetite (with a craving for carbohydrates). They gain weight, become withdrawn, sleep more and lose interest in sex. It is almost as if they go into a state of hibernation. This condition is thought to arise from high levels of the hormone melatonin in the blood stream. This hormone is secreted by the pineal gland which is situated in the head, between the under surface of the cerebrum and the mid-brain, just in front of the cerebellum (see Fig. 3).

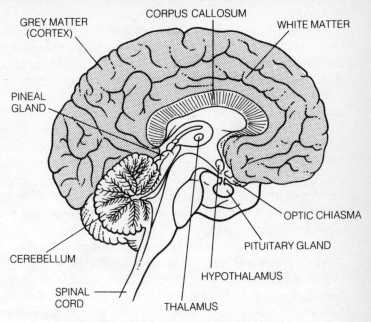

GREY MATTER
(CORTEX)

CORPUS CALLOSUM

WHITE MATTER

PINEAL
GLAND

OPTIC CHIASMA

PITUITARY GLAND

CEREBELLUM

HYPOTHALAMUS

SPINAL
CORD

THALAMUS

Fig. 3. The structure of the brain

After dark melatonin is released into the blood stream by the pineal gland. It is during the night that it reaches its highest level. During the day, especially when the sun is shining, the levels of this hormone are greatly reduced. One of the functions of the pineal gland is to act as the body's light meter and timer, synchronizing it with the seasons of the year. In the winter, with its short days and lack of sunshine, it has been discovered that people suffering from SAD have high levels of melatonin in their blood during daylight hours. This leads to the emotional disorders already described.

In 1980, Dr Alfred Lewry and Dr Thomas Wehr, discovered that bright light could suppress the normal night-time secretions of melatonin. As a result of this discovery, people with SAD were treated with bright full-spectrum light, by way of the eyes, at certain times during the day. This was found to have a beneficial effect on more than 80 per cent of those treated. This treatment is now available, but should only be administered by qualified colour therapists, and doctors who specialize in treating SAD.

Realizing how important the sun is to our well-being, and knowing that the sun has the same wave lengths as visible light, lying between 400 and 700 nanometers, it stands to reason that the radiation of visible light, made up of the eight colours of the spectrum, must affect us in a similar way.

THE HUMAN EYE AND VISIBLE LIGHT

We perceive light through our eyes, which are protected from injury by the bony sockets in which they sit. They are self-focusing, able to adapt to bright or dim light, to distant or near vision.

The eye consists of the following components: the eyeball, which is a sphere about 2.5 cms. in diameter; the sclera, which is the outer coat of the eye, seen as the white of the eye; the cornea, which is the transparent window which tends to bulge out a little; the choroid, the middle coat of the eye, composed largely of interlaced blood vessels providing nutrition to the eye; the iris, which is a continuation of the choroid and responsible for giving the eyes their colour; the pupil, the hole in the iris, which appears to be black because the inside of the eye is dark; and the retina, the innermost coat. The retina is a very thin, light-sensitive tissue which lines the back of the eye and curves forward like a deep rounded cup. The nerves from the retina join to form what is known as the optic nerve. The crystalline lens is suspended just behind the iris. The lens and its associated structure divide the eye into two compartments. The larger of these compartments is situated behind the lens and filled with a transparent liquid which ensures the eyeball maintains its correct shape; and the much smaller compartment between the cornea and lens is filled with a watery liquid (see Fig 4).

When light energy falls upon the retina, it is converted into the nerve energy that causes us to 'see'. The retina contains thousands of nerve endings which are either called 'cones' or 'rods', depending on their shape. The cones are connected individually, the rods more collectively, to cells which terminate in bunches of fibres that form the optic nerve.

Night vision is carried out by the rods which are more sensitive than the cones but which cannot distinguish colour or fine details. The cones are used in bright light and for distinguishing colour. The eye can distinguish about 7,500,000 different hues, but if a single group of colour-receptive cones is missing from the retina, an individual is unable to distinguish certain colours from others and is said to be 'colour blind'. Colour blindness is an inherited condition and affects males more frequently than females, and the most common type of colour blindness is that which makes it very difficult for a person to distinguish between red and green.

It is not only through our eyes that colour is absorbed into our being. The whole of our physical body is light sensitive, and the electromagnetic field which surrounds each one of us, is constantly filled with changing, vibrating colours. More will be said about this in a later chapter.

If we look at the design on a peacock's tail, it resembles many eyes. Our own physical body is similar to this. Each cell acts as an eye absorbing the light and colours which fall upon

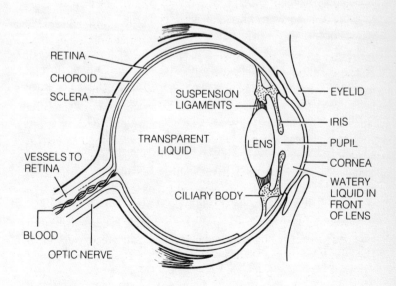

Fig. 4. A section through the eye showing the major parts

it, just as the blood stream absorbs the creams and oils which we rub into our skin.

Throughout the ages, experiments with the colours of visible light have been carried out on insects, fish, reptiles, birds and mammals, with remarkable results. It has been found that colour vision is not apparent in the lowest forms of animal life, namely the amoeba and hydra, but that it exists in insects, fish, reptiles and birds. It is lacking in most mammals, but restored again in apes and man. Scientists are largely agreed that the colour vision of insects and birds differs from that of man. In an insect, its eyes respond to the yellow region of the spectrum, but not the red; it is sensitive to green, blue, violet and ultraviolet. In birds, most are partially blind to blue but see red with remarkable clarity. In a series of experiments, a scientist named Bissonette proved that the migration and sexual cycles of birds are more dependent on light than on climatic conditions.

Working with plants, it has been found that visible light is essential for good growth and development. Plant experiments using different coloured lights have shown that their growth patterns can be greatly altered. One of the earliest investigators was Ressier of France (1783). General A. J. Pleasanton of Philadelphia who lived in the nineteenth century put forward theories which both inspired and outraged botanists of his day. One of his theories was that grapes grown under blue light become very productive in the first and second year of growth, whereas under normal light they would take five or six years to reach the same stage of production. In 1895, another researcher, C. Flammarion, claimed that plants flourished under red light. He said that this colour produced taller plants but with thinner leaves. He stated that under blue light the plant was weak and under developed. Other investigators such as L. C. Corbett (1902), Fritz Schanz (1918), H. W. Popp (1926), and S. Johnston (1936) also propounded their theories on the marked differences occuring in plants subjected to different coloured light.

A more recent investigator, Theophilus Gimbel, founder of the Hygeia College of Colour Therapy, has recorded his findings in his book *Healing Through Colour*. He asserts that experiments carried out by him show that plants grown under red light were stunted with small foliage. Green light produced brittle, weak plants, but blue light gave well-developed plants with good foliage. Perhaps each species of plant has its own reaction to the individual colours of the spectrum.

THE EIGHT COLOURS OF THE SPECTRUM

Each of the eight colours of the spectrum has its own vibrational frequency, its negative and positive attributes and its complementary colour.

In order to deepen our awareness and understanding of colour and to gain insight into why certain colours are used for some of the diseases prevalent in our society, let us examine each colour more closely. In some forms of colour therapy, the treatment colour is always used in conjunction with its complementary colour (see Fig. 5).

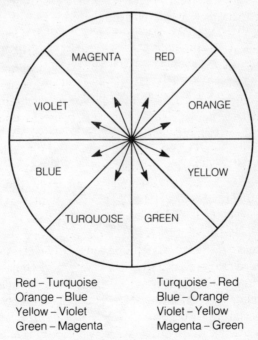

Red – Turquoise	Turquoise – Red
Orange – Blue	Blue – Orange
Yellow – Violet	Violet – Yellow
Green – Magenta	Magenta – Green

Fig. 5. Colour and complementary colour

Red

This colour has the slowest wave lengths. Like all the colours, it has its own spectrum which ranges from a very deep to a very pale red. The bright translucent shades of a colour reveal its positive aspects, whilst the dark and dingy shades reveal its negative side. As only the positive aspects are used in healing, I feel that there is no need to elaborate on the negative.

Red is the symbol of life, strength and vitality. In his book *'The Seven Keys to Colour Healing'* Ronald Hunt calls this ray the great energizer, the father of vitality. According to Hunt, red splits the ferric salt crystals into iron and salt. The red corpuscles absorb the iron, and the salt is eliminated by the kidneys and the skin. This makes it a good colour with which to treat anaemia or iron deficiency.

Red is a very powerful energizer and stimulant which I relate to the masculine energy. Through its effect on haemoglobin, it increases energy, raises body temperature and improves the circulation, which makes it a good colour for use in paralysis.

However, because of its powerful energizing and stimulating properties, red is not used a great deal in therapy, especially where there is anxiety or emotional disturbance.

When used in conjunction with its complementary colour of turquoise, red helps counteract infections. The red increases the blood supply to the area, which deals with the invading bacteria, and the turquoise helps to cleanse and reduce inflammation.

Young children love red and are attracted to it because it is a grounding and earthing colour. Until puberty, a child is establishing its roots on the earth, and red is the colour which aids this process.

Orange

Orange is the symbol of feminine energy, the energy of creation. It is more gentle than the dynamic, masculine energy of red but its energy is complementary to the red energy. It is therefore important that these two colours should work in harmony. Orange lies midway between the red and the yellow ray, and therefore influences both physical vitality and the intellect.

Orange is the colour of joy and happiness, and enables us

to create a balance between our physical and mental bodies (see Chapter 4). It gives freedom to thoughts and feelings, and disperses heaviness, allowing the body natural, joyful movements.

Orange brings about changes in the biochemical structure, resulting in the dispersing of depression. This makes it a good colour to use with people who are manic-depressive or suicidal.

The orange ray is used to treat stones in the kidney and gall bladder. Frequently these stones are caused by our own bitterness and resentment against other people or life in general. Orange has shown itself to be beneficial in cases of chronic bronchitis, and with regular treatment can clear any build-up of phlegm and the accompanying cough. Orange also has an anti-spasmodic effect and is therefore beneficial in cases of muscle spasms and cramp.

Yellow

Yellow is the symbol of the mind and intellect. It represents the power of thought and intellectuality and stimulates mental activity.

It is the colour of detachment and can help us to detach from obsessional thoughts, feelings and habits. Yellow can be an effective colour when used in conjunction with counselling because it can reveal a person's weaknesses and help to release deep-seated problems.

The yellow rays carry positive magnetic currents which are inspiring and stimulating. They strengthen the nerves and stimulate higher mentality. This colour activates the motor nerves in the physical body, thereby generating energy in the muscles. If any part of the body lacks the energy of this colour, it can manifest as partial or complete paralysis. This makes it a good colour with which to treat these conditions.

Yellow works with the skin by improving its texture, cleansing and healing scars and other disorders such as eczema. It is also used for all rheumatic and arthritic conditions because it helps to break down the calcium deposits which have formed in the joints.

Green

Green is the mid-way colour of the spectrum, being neither at the hot nor the cold end. It is the colour of balance, harmony and sympathy, and therefore has the power to bring the negative and positive energies of a human person into balance. It can also balance the three aspects of a person's being, namely body, mind and spirit, thus creating wholeness.

Green has antiseptic properties which make it useful in cases of infection. It can also be used for detoxification and in some cases of heart disease.

Experiments carried out in America by Dr William Kelly, have shown that green light destroys embryonic cell structure. He has suggested that the cancer cell is very similar in structure to the embryonic cell but, unlike the embryonic cell which follows a set genetic pattern, the cancer cell has no set pattern to follow and creates unwanted tumours in the body. In the light of this knowledge, green, with its complementary colour of magenta, is used to treat malignant tumours.

In his book *The Healing of Cancer*, Barry Lynes states that the cause of cancer was isolated by Thomas J. Glover in the 1920s as a tiny bacteria, similar in size to a virus. He continues by saying that in the middle of the 1930s, Dr W. M. Crofton of Ireland also identified the same or a similar microbe as the cause of cancer. In the light of this evidence he believes that the use of radiation, drugs and excessive surgery does not cure cancer because these methods are unable to kill the bacteria which is causing it. According to facts given in Lynes's book, Glover developed a serum which was proven to kill this bacteria, but the authorities in America refused to publish his findings.

As the result of Dr Kelly's findings that green can destroy embryonic cell structure, a pregnant woman should never be treated with this colour.

Turquoise

Turquoise is the last colour before the blue half of the spectrum, and is not normally associated with spectral colours.

Turquoise is the colour used to boost the immune system. Our immune defences against infection depend mainly on the lymphatic system. This consists of lymphatic vessels which transport tissue fluid and lymph to groups of lymph nodes, which are widely distributed throughout the body, and then into the blood stream. These lymph nodes, as well as other lymphatic tissue (for example, in the spleen, and tonsils), produce lymphocytes which have various functions; producing antibodies and attacking foreign and abnormal cells. The thymus is important in determining the character of lymphocytes, especially in early infancy and childhood, so that they do not attack the body's own tissue, but are ready to recognize and destroy invaders.

Because turquoise has a strengthening effect upon the immune system, it is used for infections, septic conditions, and AIDS. As AIDS is a virus which destroys the immune system, endeavouring to strengthen this system with turquoise can potentially prolong an AIDS sufferer's life.

Blue

This is the colour which symbolizes inspiration, devotion, peace and tranquillity. It is therefore an excellent colour to use during meditation and in places of healing.

Blue creates a sensation of space, and because of this it is said to be a cold colour. The actual temperature, however, is not influenced by the colour itself. Blue is a colour which slows things down and gives the impression of expansion. Because of this, a room painted in this colour will appear to be much larger.

It is a useful colour with which to treat tension, fear, palpitations and insomnia. Blue will reduce inflammation, and is used for laryngitis, sore throat, tonsillitis and goitres. It is also useful for shock, stings and headaches.

When blue is administered with its complementary colour, orange, it brings about a state of peaceful joy or joyful peace.

Indigo

This colour is a combination of deep blue and a small amount of red. It is not used much in healing and is therefore not included in the eight main colours of the spectrum. However, it is related to the sixth energy centre, which is discussed later in this book, and I therefore feel it is important to mention it here.

Indigo helps to broaden the mind and to free it of fears and inhibitions. Because of its relationship with the mind it can affect us psychically and also have a powerful effect on mental complaints.

Indigo is associated with the eyes and ears, and is therefore used for some diseases pertaining to these organs. Being so closely related to the blue ray, it can also help with problems related to the throat.

According to Mary Anderson, in her book '*Colour Healing*' indigo is a powerful anaesthetic and can induce complete insensitivity to pain without the loss of consciousness.

Violet

This colour pertains to spirituality, self-respect and dignity. The shining colour of violet can lift the prepared human being into a higher state of consciousness. Violet can lead us into a realm of spiritual awareness where it becomes the last gateway through which we must pass in order to become united with our true self or inner divine being.

In healing, this colour can re-strengthen a weak cell structure and restore energy. Violet is frequently needed by those who have no respect for their thoughts, feelings or physical body – the type of person who is unable to love themselves.

Violet is related to insight. It is an inspirational colour, and many of the great musicians, poets and painters have written that their moments of greatest inspiration came when they were in a predominantly violet environment.

This is a very beneficial colour for psychological disorders such as schizophrenia. It also helps sciatica, diseases of the scalp, and all disorders connected with the nervous system.

Magenta

This colour enables us to 'let go'. On a physical/mental level, it allows us to let go of ideas and thought patterns which are no longer right for us. If we hold on to ideas and conditioning which originated in our childhood and/or adolescence, we become rigid and static, no longer able to grow and evolve. This can cause frustration and fear which in due course can lead to psychological problems. Most people find it very difficult to let go and flow with the tide of life for this involves change, and change can cause feelings of insecurity and uncertainty.

In letting go and flowing with the energies of life, we no longer have a set routine or pattern. This can be very unsettling for our personality, but for our spirit it is bliss because it can move, unhindered, towards the vision which it had before it incarnated in a physical body. Once we have entered a physical body, the vision is lost to our normal senses, but the spirit remembers and will pursue it at all costs.

On the emotional level, magenta signifies letting go of feelings which are no longer relevant. Perhaps we are still trying to hold on to a relationship which we have outgrown, or maybe we are trying to relive a situation from the past. In order to learn and grow, we must emotionally let go of the past. Again, this is not easy.

When magenta fades into a very pale pink, it becomes the colour of spiritual love. This is mainly used on the emotional aspect of a person. For example, someone who is suffering from a 'broken heart' would be treated with this colour.

Magenta is the complementary colour of green which is used for malignant tumours. Sometimes I have intuitively felt that I should reverse these colours when treating a cancer patient and use magenta followed by green, and I have done this on occasion. Each human being is unique and what is the norm for 90 per cent of the population is not always the norm for the remaining 10 per cent.

Magenta can also be used in the treatment of tinnitus, benign cysts, and for detached retinas.

The information given in this chapter only provides a foundation upon which we have to build. As I have already said, each one of us is an individual, and what is regarded as the 'norm' does not always work for some individuals. This also applies in allopathic medicine – specific tablets which are prescribed for specific diseases work in the majority of cases, but for some people an alternative tablet has to be found.

Working in this particular field of complementary medicine, namely colour, we have to learn to listen to and trust our intuition. If we are able to do this when treating a patient, the correct colour will always be given.

As I have already said, colour works on all three aspects of our being – body, mind and spirit. If these three aspects are not brought into harmony, then we cannot become a whole person.

2

The History of Colour

L ET US TRAVEL back in time, as far as our memory can take
us, back into prehistory.

Prehistoric man hunted for his food, lived in caves, and
communicated in a vastly different way from present-day forms
of communication. He lived close to nature and was ruled by
her tides and seasons. For him time was governed by the phases
of the sun and moon. When light appeared with the breaking
of dawn, he worked and hunted for his food. When darkness
fell, he slept. A great deal of his time was spent in the open,
experiencing and living by the light derived from the sun.
Our present-day lifestyle is the complete opposite. Unlike
our ancestors, most of our time is spent indoors, excluding
us from the beneficial and healing natural daylight, and more
often than not subjecting us to the detrimental effects of
artificial light.

Through his close connection with nature, prehistoric man
absorbed and breathed her living colours. There is some doubt
as to whether or not he was able to 'see' colour. It is thought by
anthropologists that colour vision was not developed in prehistoric man, this faculty arising at a later stage of evolution. He
recognized that the sun was essential to life, and worshipped
her for her important role in creation.

As man evolved and developed colour vision, he associated
it with mysticism and the supernatural. He knew little about
the workings of the universe, and his survival depended upon
him living in harmony with the forces of nature. Along with
his beliefs went a great deal of superstition.

25

Since time immemorial man has gazed into the heavens, convinced that his destiny was ruled by divine forces in the sky. Over two thousand years before Christ, astrology was an important science. The seven major planets symbolized the mixture and interaction of all the essential forces of the universe and nature, and to each of these a colour was ascribed. To the sun, which sits at the centre of these planets was given the colour of gold, and to the moon which encircled the sun, silver. Black was ascribed to Saturn, orange to Jupiter, red to Mars, green to Venus, and blue to Mercury.

The use of colour is probably one of the earliest forms of therapy. Our ancestors were aware of how the colours found in nature affected them. Apart from being in close contact with the vibrations of these living colours, they absorbed colour into themselves through the food they ate.

In Atlantean times, mental, physical and emotional illness was treated with the colours which radiated from crystals. According to Frank Alpen in his three books *Exploring Atlantis* the Atlanteans built what was known as 'The Great Healing Temple'. In order to enter the temple, a person had to climb a flight of twelve steps and pass between twelve columns, six on either side. This led into a large circular room which was the heart of the temple. The ceiling of this room was domed and created out of interlocking crystals. These crystals were arranged in the form of ancient symbols which created exquisite patterns of colour when the light shone through them. Around the circumference of the room were individual healing rooms. When a patient entered one of these rooms, they were enclosed by a crystal door which was then energized to the frequency of the colour required. These rooms were not used solely for treating disease, but also for healing relationships, for childbirth, and in assisting the transition of the soul from this life to the next.

Archaeologists have discovered that the Egyptians, like the Atlanteans, had individual rooms, which were used for the purpose of healing, built into their temples. These rooms were constructed in such a way that when the sun entered them, its rays were dissipated into the colours of the spectrum. It is believed that those who came to the temple for healing were 'colour diagnosed' and then put into the room which radiated the prescribed colour. In general, the Egyptian temples were lavishly decorated with beautifully coloured drawings and hieroglyphics. Like the Ayurvedic medicine of the Indians, the Egyptians also treated with gemstones, believing them to contain the concentrated and pure colours of the universe.

THE RELIGIOUS SYMBOLISM OF COLOUR

From ancient civilizations to the present day, many cultures and religions have regarded colour as a manifestation of the Light – the divine source from which all things were created. For this reason it is ascribed to deities, is used in ceremonies, and plays an important role in mysticism and alchemy.

Black

In Indian philosophy, black is associated with the dark aspect of the Great Mother, especially with Kali (one of the names given for the consort of Shiva, pertaining to the negative aspect). The Amerindians relate black to the north and to night as opposed to the red of the day. Buddhism looks upon it as the darkness of bondage. For the Chinese, black represents the north, winter, water and, of the four spiritually endowed animals, it is affiliated to the tortoise. For Christians, black conjures up in the mind evil and hell – one of the names given to Satan is 'The Prince of Darkness'. It is the colour of mourning and the colour of a priest's vestments when worn for a requiem mass.

Unlike Christianity, the Egyptians connected this colour with rebirth and resurrection. In Hinduism, black corresponds to *Tamas*, the first of the three *gunas*, or states of being, which relates to lethargy and sensuality. Alchemists look upon black as the absence of colour and representative of the first stage of dissolution, while numerology aligns black with the number eight, and astrologers with the planet Saturn. This colour has a sinister connotation when it is connected to 'black magic' and the negative side of witchcraft.

Brown

Brown is the colour which is given to the earth and which the Hindus relate to the north. Christianity uses brown to symbolize the renunciation of the world, this being the reason some religious communities such as the Franciscans wear brown habits.

Grey

A neutral colour sometimes connected with mourning. For Christians this colour symbolizes the renunciation of the body in order to gain immortality of the soul – again, the reason why this colour is worn by certain religious communities such as the Order of the Holy Rood.

Red

In most cultures, the colour red stands for the masculine principle. It is symbolic of the sun and all the gods attributed to war. If a statue of a god is painted red, this denotes their supernatural or solar power. Red for the Amerindian means joy and fertility, and they relate it to the day as opposed to the black of the night. For Buddhists it is the colour of activity, creativity and life, known as the second *guna*, *Rajas*. The Celts have the exact opposite view of red, relating it to death and disaster. The Chinese regard it as the luckiest of all colours – for them it represents the sun, the phoenix, which is a universal symbol of resurrection and immortality, of death and rebirth by fire. In Christianity, red is the colour of martyrdom and is symbolic of the fire of Pentecost and Christ's Passion. It is a colour worn by priests for the feast days of martyrs and at Whitsuntide.

The Egyptians believed that the colour red was strongest in the autumn and in the afternoon. It is one of the colours attributed to Osiris (the other colour being green), who was originally worshipped as a nature god, embodying the spirit of vegetation which dies with the harvest and is reborn in the spring. Later he was worshipped as god of the dead.

In Greek philosophy, it is the colour given to Phoebus, the sun god, to Aries, who was the god of war, the son of Zeus and Hera and identified with the Roman god Mars. Priapus, an ancient deity personifying male generative power, was known as 'the Red God', and red is also attributed to Apollo, the Greek god of song and music to whom the famous temple at

Delphi was dedicated. The Romans related it to Mars, the god of war and husbandry; and the red poppy was sacred to Ceres, the Roman goddess of nature. Likewise, the Semitic religion associates it with Baal, the god of the sun.

Orange

The colour orange seems to have its symbolism rooted in China and Japan. These cultures look upon it as the colour of love and happiness which they show through the 'fingered citron'. The citron is one of the three blessed fruits of China, and the 'fingered citron' resembles the shape of the hand of the Buddha.

Yellow

In Buddhism, yellow is sacred, and the Buddha is sometimes depicted wearing a yellow robe. The robes worn by Buddhist monks are saffron-coloured, symbolizing renunciation, desirelessness and humility, while for Hindus a golden yellow is the colour of light, life, truth and immortality. To the Amerindian yellow signifies the west and the setting sun. The Chinese attribute yellow to the lunar hare, an animal which is given to all moon deities and which is representative of rebirth, rejuvenation, resurrection, intuition and 'light in darkness'. The hare is a *yin* animal and therefore aligned to the feminine *yin* powers.

In Christianity, yellow is linked with sacredness and divinity, and is the colour for the feast days of confessors.

Green

In Ancient Egyptian mythology, green is the alternative colour for Osiris. He was the most beloved god of the Egyptians and is said to have triumphed over death. By his resurrection he became the prototype for the faithful, and also the judge of the dead who, when justified, became one with him and thereby attained eternal life. The ceremonies connected with the celebration of the sufferings, death and resurrection of Osiris were enacted as a symbolic drama in the mystery schools of Egypt for at least five thousand years.

In Buddhism vernal green is the colour of life, while pale green depicts the kingdom of death and everything pertaining to death. The Celts attribute green to the earth goddess Bridget, and in China, green is associated with the East, wood and water. In Christianity, vernal green is the colour of immortality and hope, the growth of the Holy Spirit in man, life and the triumph over death, and the emergence of spring from winter. In medieval times it became the colour of Trinity and Epiphany. Green in the Islamic faith is a very sacred colour. Alchemists depicted green in the lion or dragon representing the beginning of the 'Great Work' the great alchemical operation and preparation for transmuting base metals into gold. Hermes Trismegistus was a great master of all arts and sciences and also a great alchemist. He is reputed to have founded the art of healing. His teachings are reported to have been written in La Table d'Emeraude (The green tablet). This text teaches that 'the thing that is on high is like the thing that is below', or 'as above so below'.

Blue

Sky blue is the colour given to the 'Great Mother', known in many religions as the 'Queen of Heaven'. In all religions it is the colour given to the gods and powers who are associated with the sky. For the Amerindian, it represents the sky and peace, while the Buddhist associates this colour with the coolness of the heavens above and the waters below. In Hinduism, Indra, the ruler of heaven, is depicted wearing a coat of blue, and to the Chinese, blue represents the heavens as well as spring and wood. In the Christian faith, it is the colour given to the Virgin Mary, the Queen of Heaven and mother of Christ. Christians relate this colour to heavenly truth and eternity. Zeus, the sky deity of Rome, who was renamed Jupiter (meaning 'father of the day') by the Romans, is represented as throned in heaven and holding in his right hand a thunderbolt, the symbol of his overlordship of the universe and of every earthly and heavenly power. His feminine counterpart, also worshipped as a sky deity, was Hera, renamed Juno by the Romans. The Romans also attributed blue to Venus, the goddess of beauty and growth in nature, whose identity was eventually merged with that of Aphrodite, through whom she assumed patronage of human love.

Purple & Violet

Purple denotes royalty and priestly power. In Christianity, it is the colour given to God the Father and is used in ceremonies and rituals throughout Lent and Advent. The Romans connected it with Jupiter, the god of thunder, rain and storm. Jupiter is also given the colour violet.

In Christianity violet is related to priestly rule and authority, and is the colour of truth, fasting and penitence. Some people purport it to be the colour of St Mary Magdelene.

Gold

God as uncreated light and divine power is symbolized by the colour gold. This colour is associated with all the sun gods, as well as the gods and goddesses pertaining to the ripening of the harvest. Its feminine principle and complementary energy is silver, the colour ascribed to the moon. To Zeus is attributed a golden cord – the cord upon which the universe is said to hang, the 'rope of heaven' upon which all things are threaded. Athena, the daughter of Zeus is reported to have worn a golden robe. In alchemy, gold is looked upon as the essence of the sun, the equilibrium of all metallic properties. The esoteric meaning of turning base metal into gold is the transmutation of the soul. The Ancient Egyptians attributed gold to the sun god Ra. For the Hindu gold means immortality, light and truth. It is the fire of Agni, the Hindu god of fire and one of the three great deities, the other two being Vayu and Surya. The colour worn by the Buddha was either yellow or gold. In the Upanishads we find written:

> . . . In the supreme golden chamber is Brahman, invisible and pure. He is the radiant light of all lights . . .

White

White is the colour from which all other colours emanate. It is the complementary energy to black. White is the colour of illumination, purity and innocence; of chastity, holiness, sacredness and redemption. The white light is symbolic of the ultimate reality, Nirvana, God-consciousness. In ancient Greece and Rome, it was the colour of mourning and this is still the case in the Orient. White can be associated with both life and love, death and burial. In the marriage ceremony, a white gown is worn to symbolize the death of an old life and the birth of a new. A white gown also stands for purity. When white is used in death, it represents the death of the physical body, making way for birth into a new life. In Christianity, white is worn at all the sacraments. It is the colour used for saints who have not been martyred, and is used at the great festivals of Easter, Christmas, Epiphany and Ascension. It denotes joy, light and innocence. The Druids wore white at baptism. For the Hindu it is the colour of pure consciousness, self-illumination and light. It is associated with the third *guna*, *Sattva*, representative of peace and the manifestation of divine truth.

In Hinduism and Christianity, the godhead has three aspects forming what is known as the Trinity. In Christianity these are: God the Father, symbolized as a hand; God the Son, symbolized by the lamb; and God the Holy Ghost, symbolized by the dove. In Hinduism, the first deity is Brahman, the creator; the second is Vishnu, the preserver; and the third is Shiva, the destroyer. Because the godhead embraces all things, and all things emanate from this being, it embraces white light. In the same way that the godhead is divided into the Trinity, so was this all pervading light. The creative power of God or Brahman, being the Father aspect, became manifest in the blue ray; the preserving and sustaining power of Vishnu and Christ the Son became manifest in the yellow ray; while Shiva, the destroyer or the disintegrating power of the Holy Ghost, is manifest in the red ray.

THE HISTORY OF COLOUR HEALING

From early civilization to the present day, countless people have researched into and worked with the healing power of colour.

At the beginning of the nineteenth century due to the discovery of new drugs and advances in surgical procedures colour therapy was temporarily replaced by allopathic medicine. Later in the same century, however, colour therapy was revived through the work of S. Pancoast and Edwin D. Babbitt.

In 1877 Pancoast published a book entitled *Blue and Red Light*, these two colours seemingly being the only ones he used. He treated by passing light through panes of red and blue glass, the rays of which were focused on to his patient. According to his records, his treatments were frequently successful.

Edwin Babbitt received recognition when his book *The Principles of Light and Colour* was published in 1878. His treatment differed from that of Pancoast in that he used yellow light in addition to red and blue. For the transmission of colour, he developed a cabinet which made use of natural sunlight, and which he called the 'Thermoline'. This was later remodelled so that the source of light came from what he described as an 'electric arc'. With this new cabinet he used a 'chromo disc' to which he fitted coloured filters which were able to localize the required colour on to the part of the body where it was needed. He is also reported to have used solarized water in his treatments. For solarizing water, he hung in the sunlight a small glass bottle fitted with a 'chromo lens' (which he developed for this purpose) of the colour required. This water was then given to the patient to drink.

In 1934, Dinshah P. Ghadiali published his three-volume work, the *Spectro-Chrome Metry Encyclopedia*, which constituted a home training course. He believed that sound, light, colour, magnetism and heat were all the same energy, the only difference being their vibrational frequency. He related colour and vibration to the physiology of the body, believing that no elements are pure but that the elements themselves are compounds which do not possess a single or pure spectrum. He invented two machines which transmitted colour through slides. The first, which he called the 'graduate spectro-chrome', contained a 2,000-watt concentrated bulb, was driven by a motor and had built into it revolving coloured slides which were housed in an aluminium slide carrier. The second machine was the aluminium spectro-chrome which he invented for the family. This contained a 1,000-watt bulb and a sealed semaphore slide carrier which contained the

Dinshah attuned colour wave slides. It had its own stand and an automatic time switch, and came complete with a spectro-chrome home guide.

In volume 3 of the *Spectro-Chrome Metry Encyclopedia*, Ghadiali writes:

> In its reparative, recuperative and rejuvenative processes the Human Body is subject to certain Laws Of Periodicity. These hitherto unknown Laws, were first discovered and applied by the Originator of Spectro-Chrome Metry. The great success in the use of Spectro-Chrome depends on a definite application of these Laws, which are partly Astronomical, partly Gravitational, partly Physiological and above all Radiational. They are exceedingly intricate and difficult to realize, but I simplified the complicated procedure by codifying all the laws pertaining to the variations.

Back in 1666 Isacc Newton had discovered, by the use of a prism, that all the colours exist in solar light and can be separated from each other through refraction. This was refuted in the nineteenth century by Goethe who wrote *The Theory of Colour*. Unlike his predecessors in this field, Goethe believed that colour was a living entity. His theory of colour differed from Newton's in that he saw colours arising through the interplay of light and dark. He also believed that there was a spiritual significance behind colour which had been overlooked by his contemporaries, and it was Goethe's work which provided the foundation for Rudolph Steiner's work on colour.

Steiner (1861–1925) has been regarded as an occultist, philosopher, teacher and religious leader. He was the founder of the anthroposophical society and in 1919 founded the Waldorf Schools which were later named the Rudolf Steiner Schools. He was reputed to be far advanced in his theory of colours and predicted that colour therapy would play an important role in the coming age. He believed that illness was caused through the separation of earthly consciousness from higher perception and that this could be healed through art. He divided colours into two categories. These were the colours of activity: red, blue and yellow; and the image colours: green, white, black and peach blossom which he related to form.

In his book *'New Light on the Eyes'*(1958) E. Brooke Simpkins purported that eyes need the energy of light in the same way that the body needs food. He believed that the therapeutic value of colour is particularly potent when applied through the eyes, and in his book he claims to have successfully treated cataracts by shining the appropriate coloured light into the eyes.

A modern-day researcher into the importance of light to the eyes is Jacob Liberman. In his book *Light, Medicine of the Future*, he discusses the therapeutic use of light and colour in the treatment of various cancers, depression, stress, visual problems, PMS, the human immune system, and learning disabilities. Like the pioneers of heliotherapy, he also believes that sunlight is vital to our well-being.

Through the work of these people and those of us who are still researching into colour, more knowledge is being gained about the wonderful healing powers of visible light. How this knowledge can be used to benefit humanity is discussed in a later chapter.

MEDITATION AND COLOUR

Through meditation I have experienced colours which are not seen on the earth plane. Because as yet they have not become manifest on the earth plane and we can therefore only see them with our 'inner eyes', it is impossible to describe them – our language is inadequate for this higher realm.

Some people have tried to experience and touch this higher realm through the use of drugs, and drug taking played an important role in almost every primitive religion. The Greeks, Persians and the ancient Hindus, for example, used alcohol to produce religious ecstasy. The Mexicans tried to gain this state of bliss by taking an intoxicant called *peyote*, which was made from cactus tops and contained mescaline. It was used mainly in religious ceremonies. Drug-induced ecstasy is still an essential part of the religious rituals of many African, South American and Polynesian peoples, and in the West we are aware of the use of the psychedelic drug, LSD, in our society.

In his books *The Doors of Perception* and *Moksha*, Aldous Huxley describes the results of the clinical tests which he carried out with mescalin, LSD and *Amanita muscaria* (more commonly known as the 'Sacred Mushroom'), in order to learn about and experience this state of ecstasy. He points out that all drugs have side effects and can be addictive. The other problem with taking hallucinatory drugs is that one does not always reach this ecstatic state but can experience what some users of LSD have described as a 'bad trip'. When drugs were used in religious ceremonies, the people taking them made sure that their bodies were pure and free from toxins. This entailed certain religious observances, including fasting. Drugs may seem a 'short cut' into this higher realm, but the risks to oneself are high. Meditation may take much longer and require discipline from the meditator, but the risks are minimal and the benefits great.

Sound has a very special relationship to colour and we can introduce colour into our body through mantra meditation, which uses sound. The well-known mantra AUM is akin to the sacred number three: the letter A symbolizes the conscious or waking state, the letter U the dream state, and the letter M the dreamless sleep state. The entire word, encompassing the crescent and the dot (see Fig. 6.), stands for the fourth state which in Sanskrit is known as *Samadhi* and which relates to the colour white. (In Hinduism *Samadhi* is known as *Nirvana*, and in Christianity as God-consciousness.) The letters in the word 'AUM' also represent the triad of Divinity: 'A' is Brahma the creator, and relates to blue; 'U' is Vishnu the preserver, relating to yellow, and 'M' is Shiva the destroyer, relating to red. Putting the individual sounds together into 'AUM' enables each individual consciousness to be lifted into the white light of God-consciousness which embraces the 'All'.

The three letters are also representative of the dimensions of length, breadth and depth, while the entire symbol represents Divinity which is beyond the limitations of shape and form and which manifests as white light. The letters correspond to the three tenses, past, present and future while the entire symbol stands for the creator who transcends the limitations of time.

There are many sacred words used in mantra meditation, and each person has either to be given the sound which is right for them (as in Transcendental Meditation), or find the right sound themselves. But whichever sound is used, like AUM, it is linked to the vibrations of colour.

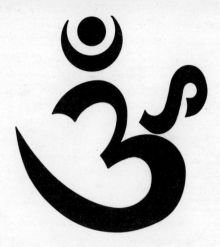

Fig. 6. The symbol of 'OM' (AUM)

There are many ways of meditating, and each individual should explore all of them and then choose the one which is most beneficial. It is wise to be taught meditation from one who is experienced in this art rather than to teach oneself from books. There is a saying in yoga: 'When the student is ready the master will appear.' This is equally true for meditation. If a person is a true seeker, then he will find what he needs.

As we enter fully into this New Age, I believe that the planet earth and its occupants will be raised into a higher vibrational frequency. This will bring with it an expansion of consciousness. With this will come the responsibility which is needed in order for us to 'see', experience and work with these as yet unmanifested colours. It has been predicted that colour and sound will be the medicine of the future. I am sure that for some people this sounds a little like science fiction. For others, it is already a reality. Aldous Huxley, through his experiments, concluded that 'Colour is the very touchstone of reality'. I believe that colour is a force of immeasurable and infinite power and is the living language of light.

3

How Does Colour Therapy Work?

EACH OF US is made up of body, mind and spirit and in order to become a whole person, these three aspects have to be brought into harmony.

We are all aware that we have a physical body. It is the tangible part of us, the part we can touch. We also acknowledge the mind, some people being better able to control this than others. But when we mention the spiritual part of our being, we find there are people who would like to believe in this aspect of themselves, those who half believe in it, and those who completely dismiss it. On the other hand, there are the few for whom it has become a reality.

Coming back to our physical body, most people have some idea of how it is made up and how it works. They may not comprehend its functions in detail but they know that it consists of a skeletal system which is supported and made mobile by muscles. They appreciate that inside the torso are organs which constitute the various systems of the body – such as the digestive, circulatory, respiratory, reproductive, and immune systems – all of which work in perfect harmony when given the right conditions. Covering the outside of the body is the skin which is waterproof and covered with tiny hairs which act as antennae. The whole of the physical body is composed of cells which are constantly dying and being replaced; and a large percentage of the body is fluid which makes it subject to the phases of the moon.

The physical body is a living organism, and as such is constantly changing and moving, even though we think that we are sitting or standing still. This constant movement sets up a vibrational frequency which differs for each organ, muscle, gland, bone and skin, and which is unique to each individual. These vibrational frequencies are akin to the vibrational frequencies of the many shades of the eight major colours we have already discussed. These frequencies can also be attuned to sound, and when this is done the individual becomes a symphony of modulating harmonies. If a person becomes ill, we can liken them to an instrument going out of tune. At the same time, the colours which radiate from the body either become a dingy, murky shade of the original colour or change into a completely different colour. The principle of colour therapy is to administer the colour or colours which the sick person is lacking, in order to retune and bring their body back into harmony.

If the body has become diseased, there must be a cause. Unless the cause is found and worked with, no matter how many times one 'retunes' the body with colour it will repeatedly go out of tune. An example which I frequently give is of someone hitting their head against a wall. No matter how much arnica is applied to the bruising, it will not be healed unless the person stops hitting their head against the wall. When a person attends for colour therapy, we try to find the cause through counselling. Once the cause has been uncovered, only the patient can resolve it, for as individuals, we are the only people who can be responsible for our own lives and bodies.

THE AURA

Apart from our physical body, we also have a subtle body surrounding us which is known as the aura or electromagnetic field. The size of this varies with each individual, depending upon their spiritual awareness – the aura of the Buddha is reported to have extended for three miles!

The aura is ovoid in shape, the widest part being near the head and the smallest near the feet (see Fig. 7).

The aura is made up of six sheaths or layers, all of them interpenetrating each other and the physical body. There are six layers which constitute the subtle body: the etheric

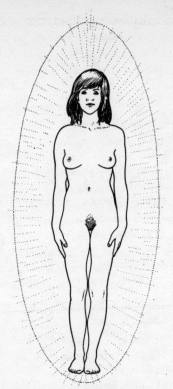

Fig. 7. The aura

or energy body which extends about two inches from the physical body; the astral or emotional body; the mental body; the higher mental body; the causal body; and the bodyless body. Each of these subtle bodies contains energy centres or *chakras* radiating colours which mingle and penetrate each other, thereby filling the aura with a cascade of ever-changing rainbows. The colours in the etheric sheath are quite dense, but as we pass through the other layers the colours emanated by their respected chakras become much finer and ethereal. As I have already said, these colours change with our moods and health patterns.

The Bodyless Body

Taking each of these layers separately, the bodyless body is referred to by many religions as the 'divine spark' or the 'true essence' — the eternal or spiritual part of us which will eventually return to God or the cosmic ocean of consciousness. Many people find this theory very difficult to grasp. In the Chandogya Upanishad it is described thus:

> Svetaketu Aruneys, a boy who was proud of his knowledge of sacred wisdom, was asked by his father if he knew about the spiritual, eternal essence which was contained in all beings. The boy said that he did not and asked his father to teach him. The father said: 'Believe me my son, an invisible and subtle essence is the spirit of the whole universe. That is Reality. That is Atman. *Thou art that.*'
>
> 'Explain more to me, father,' said Svetaketu.
>
> 'So be it my son. Place this salt in water and come to me tomorrow morning.'
>
> Svetaketu did as he was commanded, and in the morning his father said to him: 'Bring me the salt you put into the water last night.'
>
> Svetaketu looked into the water but could not find it, for it had dissolved.
>
> His father then said: 'Taste the water from this side. How is it?'
>
> 'It is salt.'
>
> 'Taste it from the middle. How is it?'
>
> 'It is salt.'
>
> 'Taste it from that side. How is it?'
>
> 'It is salt.'
>
> 'Look for the salt again and come to me.'
>
> The son did so saying: 'I cannot see the salt, I only see water.'
>
> His father then said: 'In the same way, O my son, you cannot see the spirit, but in truth he is here. An invisible and subtle essence is the spirit of the whole universe. That is Reality. That is Truth. *Thou art that.*'

For many of my yoga students, this story has made this reality much easier to understand.

The Causal Body

The next sheath is the casual body. This contains the record of our previous incarnations – the lessons we have learnt, and the experience and knowledge we have mastered. It also contains the cause or reason why we have incarnated into our present life. When we choose to incarnate into a physical body, we choose the parents and the environment which will give us the experiences that we need in order to evolve and grow nearer to out source of origin. We also know what our tasks and challenges are for the life span which we have chosen. Unfortunately, from the minute we are born we are subject to conditioning which makes us forget our plan. We then become like travellers working our way across strange country without a map. Sometimes, in moments of silence, we are given insight and inspiration which helps us forward. These are rememberings from the causal body which have managed to filter through to our conscious mind via the higher mental body. When, after many incarnations and through discipline, a person is able to identify with the divine spark within, then they are able to recall past lives at will.

The Higher Mental Body

The fifth sheath, the higher mental body, is where our intuition lies. It is through this body that we are able to communicate, be inspired and taught by the masters who have walked the earth and are now in the world of spirit. It is also where our own true divine self is able to instruct and guide us. For seventy-five per cent of the population, these higher sheaths or levels of consciousness are undeveloped. The best way to gently work with them is through guided meditation and by following a spiritual discipline. This normally happens at the exact moment when an individual is ready to move forward.

The Mental Body

The fourth layer, the mental body, is where thought patterns accumulate. Each thought that we think creates a pattern or form. These accumulate in the mental body and can be projected out into the environment, surrounding us with thought forms which we and other individuals have created. If we think unkind thoughts about another person, we project these thoughts in form shapes to that person. The more powerful the thought, the more damage it can do. These thought forms also attract the thought forms surrounding us which are of a similar nature. Therefore, if we think negative thoughts we will attract negative thought forms; likewise, positive thoughts attract positive thought forms. From this, we can see how important it is to stand back and look at what we are thinking and if it is at all negative, to change it into something positive. This is far from easy, but with a little practice it can be achieved. There is a lovely story of the Buddha being in the presence of a person who was mentally throwing daggers at him. When they reached his aura, he changed them into beautiful flowers before sending them back.

The Astral Body

The third sheath is the astral or emotional body. In most people this is frequently in a state of imbalance as they allow their emotions to rule them – one day they may be full of the joys of spring, and the next be depressed and miserable. In yoga, this is likened to the pendulum on a clock, constantly swinging from left to right from joy to despair. If we can learn to climb up the pendulum to the point where it is attached to the clock, we will experience equilibrium because it is at this point that all movement ceases. In other words, it is here that we can learn to detach from our emotions in order to see them for what they really are.

People who are highly emotional create a great deal of stress in their body. This prevents the body from functioning at its full potential and subsequently it becomes dis-eased. (It is well known, for example, that stomach ulcers are strongly related to emotional stress.

The Etheric Body

The sheath nearest to the physical body is the etheric. The etheric and physical body are very closely interwoven and disintegrate together at death. Every physical particle has its etheric counterpart which is a perfect replica of the physical form. This is why it is known as the etheric double, and why people who have had a limb amputated can still feel pain or sensation from it – it is still present in its etheric form. The etheric lays down the basic pattern upon which the physical body is built. This means that the resilience of the physical body is directly related to the tone and quality of the etheric body. To the clairvoyant, the etheric body resembles a luminous web of fine bright lines of force known as *nadis*. In a healthy person, these stand at right angles to the physical body, but in a person who is ill or tired and depleted of energy these lines are seen to droop, similar to a plant in need of water. The three main nadis are the central channel, the *sushumna*, *pingala* on the right and *ida* on the left. *Ida* and *pingala* start at the base chakra at the base of the spine, and move around each chakra in an upward spiral until they terminate at the brow chakra. The pattern which they make is that of the caduceus, the symbol used by the medical profession (see Fig. 8).

The most important function of the etheric body is the transference of life energy from the universal field via the etheric body to the physical body. This life force is known as *prana*. On a bright sunny day *prana* is in abundance and can be seen as minute glowing particles in the atmosphere. *Prana* is the reason we feel good when the sun shines.

THE CHAKRAS

The transference of *prana* takes place through the seven main energy centres or chakras which are situated along the etheric spine. These force centres can be found in each of the six layers constituting the aura, but their primary importance is at the etheric level. They are both the transformers and the transmitters of energy for each of the layers. In appearance they resemble a wheel, the Sanskrit word *chakra* meaning a wheel or circle. The energies rhythmically pulsate and circulate through the core of this wheel, and resemble the petals of a flower. In Indian philosophy, the chakras are likened to lotus flowers, and the number of petals given to each flower is in alignment with its energies. These centres are never still, but the speed with which they rotate depends

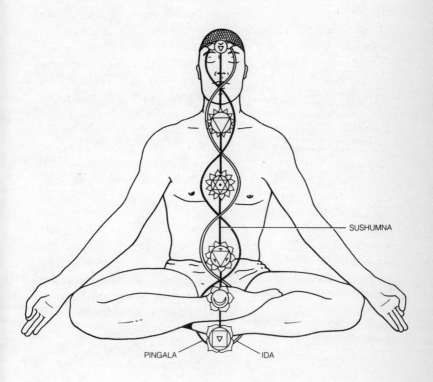

Fig. 8. The three main nadis

to some extent upon the state of health of the individual (see Fig. 9).

Five of the major chakras in the etheric body are in alignment with the spine, while the sixth and seventh are located between the eyebrows and just above the crown of the head, respectively. The size of these centres is related to an individual's personal development. In an undeveloped person the chakras will be small in size, slow in movement and dull in colour. In a more intelligent and sensitive person,

45

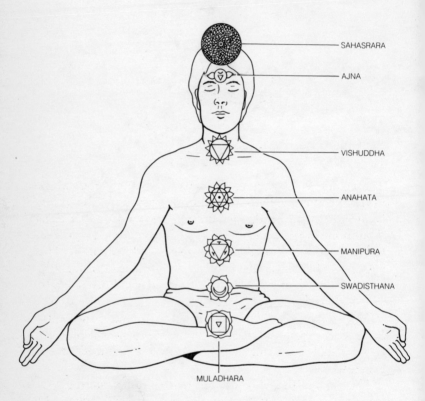

SAHASRARA

AJNA

VISHUDDHA

ANAHATA

MANIPURA

SWADISTHANA

MULADHARA

Fig. 9. The seven major chakras

they will be larger in size, faster in movement, and brighter in colour. In a newborn baby, the chakras are about three centimetres across.

To each of these centres is ascribed a dominant colour, and each centre has a special link with one of the endocrine glands and with certain physical organs. In order to understand the importance of these centres and their associated endocrine glands, let us look at each one in turn.

The Base Centre

The base centre or muladhara chakra is situated at the end of the coccyx. It is symbolized by a deep red lotus flower with four petals.

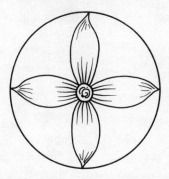

The colour which radiates from it is red, the colour which in the spectrum vibrates at the lowest frequency. This centre is said to contain the primal energy, known as the *kundalini shakti*. One of the aims of yoga is to raise this energy in order to bring about a state of enlightenment and realization. This must never be undertaken lightly. When a person is mentally, physically and spiritually ready, this energy will rise naturally and safely to his or her benefit.

This chakra is associated with the earth, and is the centre of physical energy and vitality. It regulates the sense of smell, is associated with will and power, and is ascribed to the planet Mars.

The parts of the body affected by this centre are the legs, feet, bones, large intestine, spine, and nervous system. The endocrine glands to which it is related are the gonads. These constitute the testes in the male, and the ovaries in the female.

The hormones secreted from the testes are called androgens, the most important being testerone which is responsible for the changes which take place in a male during puberty.

Apart from producing ova, the ovaries, secrete oestrogen and progesterone. The secretion of oestrogen is influenced by the follicle-stimulating-hormone (FSH) which is produced by the pituitary gland. Oestrogen helps to regulate the menstrual cycle and develops the sexual characteristics of the female.

Progesterone sensitizes the mucous membrane of the uterus in preparation for the fertilized ovum.

When this centre is functioning fully, it gives a person a strong will to live on the physical plane. He/she is filled with vitality and energy, nothing is too much trouble, and the whole of life becomes an adventure. If, however, this centre is blocked, the person's energy levels will be low, they will have no enthusiasm for life, and will feel unable to carry out their daily work.

The Swadisthana or Sacral Centre

Swadisthana is a Sanskrit word meaning 'one's own abode'. It is situated halfway between the pubis and the navel, and it is symbolized by an orange lotus flower with six petals. In yoga these six petals are likened to states of consciousness: credulity, suspicion, disdain, delusion, false knowledge, and pitilessness.

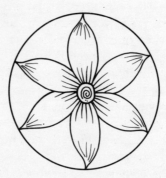

Swadisthana is associated with the element water, and affects the flow of fluids in the body, and the dominant colour which it radiates is orange. The orange energy is of a much finer quality than the 'down-to-earth' energy of the base centre. It is associated with sex and does not awaken until puberty. Swadisthana has an affinity with the throat centre, and in certain *tantric* practices and disciplines, the sexual energy from this centre can be transmuted to the throat centre where it is used for creativity and communication. (Tantra yoga is a spiritual science which involves techniques by which a person can enter the sub-conscious and unconscious mind. These methods are also aimed at awakening the powerful energy in man, known in yoga as the kundalini force, in order that man may realize his true or divine self which is eternal.)

This centre links with the emotions of fear and anxiety. The glands and organs which it influences are the skin, the reproductive organs (especially in the female), the kidneys, bladder, circulatory system, and lymphatic system. The endocrine glands associated with it are the adrenals.

Each human being has two adrenal glands, one on the top of each kidney. They are approximately one inch in length and yellowish in colour. They constitute an outer cortex and an interior or medulla. The hormones secreted by the cortex are influenced by the hormone adrenocorticotrophin (ACTH) which is secreted by the pituitary gland.

The cortex is responsible for secreting a number of hormones known as corticosteroids. These are divided into three main groups: The first group are the mineral corticoids. These work on the tubules of the kidneys, helping to retain sodium and chloride in the body, maintaining blood pressure and aiding in the excretion of excess potassium.

The second group are called gluco-corticoids, the most important being hydrocortisone (cortisol). These assist in the conversion of carbohydrates into glycogen. They increase the blood sugar, help in the utilization of fat, decrease the number of lymphocytes and eosinophils in the blood, and reduce the rate at which certain connective tissue cells multiply. In excess this action tends to suppress natural healing and therefore delays it.

The third group are similar to the hormones produced by the gonads. They influence the growth and sex development in both male and female.

The medulla of the adrenal glands secretes adrenalin and nor-adrenalin. Adrenalin stimulates the sympathetic nervous system and causes the arteries of the body to constrict, resulting in an increase in the heartbeat and a rise in blood pressure. Adrenalin also stimulates the liver into converting glycogen into glucose which it then pours into the bloodstream. Nor-adrenalin is a related substance which increases blood pressure and heart rate.

When this centre is blocked, it can result in a woman being unable to reach orgasm during sexual union. In a male it manifests as premature ejaculation or the inability

to achieve an erection. Other disorders which can be caused
are abnormalities in the kidney and bladder functions, such
as infections and poor urinary control, and problems with
the circulatory system, menstruation and the production of
seminal fluids.

When this centre is functioning to its full potential, it opens
the intuitive and psychic powers. When it first awakens, it can
upset the sexual energies and heighten awareness to external
stimuli. These will again find their own balance but on a higher
level of consciousness.

The Manipura or Solar Plexus Chakra

This centre is situated between the twelfth thoracic and the
first lumbar vertebrae. It is depicted as a bright yellow lotus
flower with ten petals.

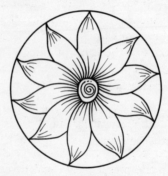

The word *manipura*, means 'city of jewels' or 'filled with
jewels'. This centre is so called because it is the fire centre,
the focal point of heat which radiates like a golden sun. It is
ruled by the sun and is associated with active intelligence.

In Chinese philosophy, this centre is called the 'triple
warmer' because during the process of digestion heat is
generated. In the teachings of the Japanese, it is called the
Hara, which means belly.

This is the centre of vitality in the psychic and physical
bodies because it is the centre where *prana* (the upward-
moving vitality) and *apana* (the downward-moving vitality)
meet, generating the heat that is necessary to support life.
When these two energies join, the centre awakens.

On an emotional level, this chakra plays an important role. This is mainly due to the fact that the astral energy enters the etheric field at the solar plexus. In most people, this chakra is the most active of all because it is involved in emotional life. It is most active in a person with strong desires and emotions.

At a physical level, this centre is chiefly concerned with the process of digestion and absorption. The processes and organs influenced by it are the breath, the diaphragm, stomach, duodenum, gall bladder and liver. The endocrine gland with which it is associated is the pancreas.

The pancreas is situated behind the stomach, and lies transversely across the posterior abdominal wall at the level of the first and second lumbar vertebrae. This gland is similar in structure to the salivary glands which are found in the mouth.

Only part of the pancreas is endocrine. These are the 'islets of Langerhans' which secrete insulin, which is responsible for the metabolism of sugar. Without insulin, the muscles would be unable to use the sugar which circulates in the blood. Sugar is used by the tissues in the form of glucose, and in order to produce energy, this is broken down into carbon dioxide and water. Any excess sugar in the blood is stored in the liver as glycogen.

If the islets of Langerhans are not functioning properly, there will be a lack of insulin which will result in diabetes, a condition in which the blood sugar is too high. It is normally diagnosed through the presence of sugar in the urine.

When this chakra is unstable, a person can be subjected to rapid mood swings. There will be a tendency towards depression, introversion, lethargy, poor digestion, and abnormal eating habits. Its malfunction can lead to nervous instability and to cancer, if the energies from the heart centre fail to be expressed on the physical plane. This centre interacts between the heart and the sacral centre, and if it is blocked, sexuality cannot be connected to love. When this centre is open, a deep and fulfilling emotional life is experienced.

This centre is also related to inner connectedness. When two people enter into a friendship, cords are formed between the solar plexus of each – the stronger the relationship, the stronger the cords. If the relationship ends, the cords are slowly disconnected. A similar cord is formed between a mother and her newborn child.

The Anahata or Heart Centre

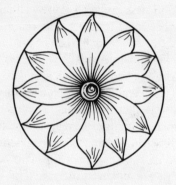

This chakra is situated between the fourth and fifth thoracic vertebrae, and is symbolized by a green lotus flower with twelve petals. When the colour radiating from this centre is clear with a steady rhythm it is indicative of a healthy heart. It is associated with the element of air and the sense of touch. Its ruling planet is Venus and it is associated with the quality of harmony through conflict.

The word *anahata* means the 'unstruck'. All the sound in the universe is produced by striking objects together. This sets up vibrations or sound waves. The primordial sound, which comes from beyond this world, is the source of all sound. This is the centre where the sound manifests.

On a physical level, anahata is associated with the heart and circulatory system, the lungs and respiratory system, the immune system, and the arms and hands. The endocrine gland attributed to it is the thymus.

The thymus gland is situated in the thorax, behind the sternum and in front of the heart. It consists mainly of lymphoid tissue and plays a part in the formation of lymphocytes. At birth this gland is quite large and continues to increase in size until puberty, at which point it starts to shrink. The thymus plays an important part in the body's immune system by producing thymus-derived lymphocy. It is claimed that through certain yogic practices this gland can be kept active, thereby keeping a person youthful and the immune system strong.

This is the centre through which we love. Love can be expressed on many levels. It can be purely selfish, demanding and constricting, or it can be compassionate and caring. The more open this centre is, the greater our capacity to extend undemanding spiritual love. When a person has transformed personal desires and passions into a love which encompasses his fellow human beings, animals and nature, the energies from the solar plexus are raised into this centre. It is through this centre that we make cords to connect with those with whom we have a love relationship. When this centre is open, we can perceive the beauty and spiritual love in our fellow human beings. Its awakening brings a greater sensitivity to touch, and a detachment from material objects.

This centre is linked with the crown chakra and the dimensions of higher consciousness. This link can be strengthened through the practice of meditation.

The Vishuddha or Throat Chakra

The word *vishuddha* means to purify, hence this chakra is the centre of purification. It is symbolized by a smoky violet blue lotus with sixteen petals. It is connected with the planet mercury, and is associated with concrete science and knowledge.

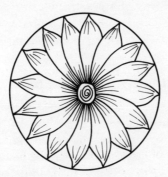

The throat centre is purported to be the place where divine nectar (the mystical elixir of immortality) is tasted. This nectar is a kind of sweet secretion produced by the gland known as the *lalana chakra* which is located near the back of the throat. This nectar gland is stimulated by higher yogic practices, and it is claimed that the nectar can sustain a yogi for any length of time without food or water.

On the physical level, this chakra governs the nervous system, the female reproductory organs, the vocal cords, and the ears. The endocrine glands associated with it are the thyroid and parathyroids.

The thyroid gland is situated in the lower part of the neck. It consists of two lobes, which are positioned on either side of the trachea and joined by an isthmus which passes in front of the trachea. The active hormones of this gland are thyroxine and triodothyronine. Iodine is an important element in these hormones. Their main function is to regulate the rate of metabolic processes in the body, and they are necessary for normal growth and development, particularly in childhood. They keep the skin and hair in good condition and co-operate with other ductless glands to keep the endocrine balance in the body.

The parathyroids are situated behind each of the four poles of the thyroid gland. They are about the size of a pea and secrete the hormone parathormone, which controls the calcium metabolism of the body.

The throat centre is the creative centre, especially of the spoken word. In singers and people who practise public speaking this centre is larger than average, brighter and faster moving. This centre is sensitive to colour, sound and form, and therefore very alive in anyone who is connected with creativity in any of its many manifestations.

The Ajna or Brow Chakra

The word *ajna* means 'command' and it is at this centre that one receives commands from the higher self. It is situated at the centre of the brow, and is composed of ninety-six petals but depicted by just two petals. This may be because this chakra appears to clairvoyants as being divided into two segments. It is the centre of visualization and perception, and reflects the twofold nature of the mind – the ego self and the spirit self, the reasoning mind and the intuitive mind. The mind can be focused on higher, spiritual ideals or on the mundane world. At this centre the two main nadis, the *ida* (masculine) and the *pingala* (feminine) meet. Thus it is at this centre that the feminine and masculine aspects of a person merge into one, bringing about a spiritual awakening.

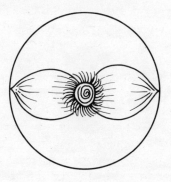

On the physical level it is related to the eyes, nose, ears and brain. The endocrine gland with which it is associated is the pituitary.

The pituitary gland is about one centimetre in diameter and is situated at the base of the brain. It consists of an anterior and posterior lobe, both having different modes of development and entirely different functions.

The anterior lobe of the pituitary gland is frequently referred to as the master gland of the endocrine system. The reason for this is that its hormonal secretions control the activities of the other endocrine glands. The many hormones which it secretes are under the influence of the hypothalamus.

The posterior lobe secretes two hormones: vasopressin which is an antidiuretic hormone; and oxytocin which stimulates the lactating breast to effect milk, and stimulates the plain muscles of the uterus during and immediately after labour.

Instability in this centre leads to tiredness, irritability, confusion and rigid thoughts. Imbalances can also lead to sinus problems, catarrh, hay fever, sleeplessness, mental stress, neuritis and migraine.

The Sahasrara Chakra

The sahasrara chakra is situated just above the crown of the head. It consists of twelve golden central petals which are surrounded by nine hundred and sixty secondary petals, and is therefore called the 'thousand-petalled lotus'. The predominant colour is violet.

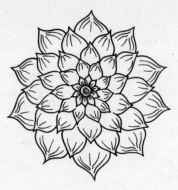

A thousand is the number which represents infinity. This chakra leads us into the eternal, infinite, supreme existence. It is the centre of pure consciousness. This centre is ruled by the planet Neptune and is associated with ceremonial white magic. The endocrine gland with which it is associated is the pineal.

The pineal gland is a small reddish-grey structure about the size of a pea. It is situated between the under surface of the cerebrum and the mid-brain, just in front of the cerebellum. Its main secretion is melatonin which affects the body's biological clock. The level of melatonin in the blood is highest at night, gradually decreasing during the daylight hours. This gland regulates the onset of puberty, induces sleep, and influences our moods.

When this centre is open, a person sees his/her spirituality in a very personal way – a spirituality that is not tied up with any dogma.

Minor Chakras

Apart from the seven major chakras, the body contains twenty-one minor and numerous smaller chakras, these being the points used in acupuncture.

From the knowledge and understanding of these centres of energy, the colours which radiate from them, and their association with the physical body, we can begin to understand how important it is that they are kept in a state of harmony and balance. If they are not, then eventually the imbalance will manifest as disease in the physical body. Part of a colour therapy treatment involves working with the etheric or energy body and balancing the chakras, while the rest of the treatment is made up of treating the physical body, and counselling. Carrying out a colour therapy treatment in this way works not only with the physical and etheric aspects, but also with the mental, emotional and spiritual aspects of the patient. This treatment will be explained in the next chapter.

4

How Colour is Used in Therapy

THERE ARE MANY ways in which colour can be used in therapy. From the previous chapters you will have discovered how the pioneers in this field created and built instruments, and formulated ways to transmit colour to their patients. Some of these techniques have become obsolete, whilst others, with varying degrees of modification, have stood the test of time.

One way frequently used to transmit colour is by passing light through coloured filters. Through trial and error, it has been discovered that the best material to use here is stained glass. Unlike plastic gels which are used by some practitioners, stained glass contains the complete vibrational spectrum of its given colour. This enables a person to absorb the correct shade and vibration of the colour needed to bring the body back into harmony.

When working with colour in this way, it has proved beneficial to use the prescribed colour in conjunction with its complementary colour (see Fig. 5 on p. 17). The reason for this is that the combination of the colours stabilizes the condition. Take for example the treatment of high blood pressure. A person treated for this condition only with blue, showed an initial lowering of their blood pressure, but a short time after treatment it rose again to a dangerously high level. The same condition was then treated with blue together with its complementary colour orange. This time the blood pressure fell, but then remained stable after treatment.

METHODS OF COLOUR DIAGNOSIS

In order to be able to treat a person with colour, a means has to be adopted whereby the required colour can be ascertained. There are several ways of doing this, some of which are very simple whilst others are more complex but render a great deal more information.

Two simple ways of finding the treatment colour are kinesiology and dowsing.

Applied Kinesiology

Applied kinesiology is based on special muscle testing techniques through which weaknesses are identified and treated, thereby correcting imbalances in the body's energy system. When this method is used to determine which colour is needed, the patient holds up each of the colours of the spectrum in turn at eye level with their left hand. Meanwhile, their right arm is held horizontal to the body. As each colour is looked through, the therapist applies gentle downward pressure to the patient's right arm. If there is no resistance to this pressure, it indicates that the person needs the colour which they are holding.

Dowsing

When used in healing, dowsing is normally performed with a pendulum on a length of string. By relaxing the mind, a person is able to contact their intuition or higher self and receive answers – in the form of 'yes' or 'no' – through the movement of the pendulum. Before working with this method, the operator must learn the specific response of the pendulum to their 'yes' or 'no'. This can take various forms such a clockwise or anti-clockwise rotation, or a vertical or horizontal swing. Once this art has been mastered, it can be very accurate.

Dowsing can be traced back to shamanism. When a shaman experienced difficulty in entering into communication with the spirits, or when the spirit messages were unclear, he would employ a primitive form of pendulum, a pebble hung on a thread. He would then ask it questions. The way the pendulum moved in response to these questions, whether back and forth or sideways, clockwise or anti-clockwise, provided him with the answers. When using this method to find the appropriate colour, the therapist lists the eight colours and asks which one is needed.

Colour Diagnostic Chart

One of the more complex methods employs a colour diagnostic chart. This method is taught at the Hygeia College of Colour Therapy.

The diagnostic chart (see Fig. 10) shows the thirty-two vertebrae of the human spine, and these vertebrae are divided into four sections of eight. To the eight vertebrae in each of the four sections is attributed one of the colours of the spectrum. Starting from the cervical part of the spine and working downwards to the coccyx, the first eight vertebrae constitute the mental aspect of a person; the second section constitutes the emotional aspect; the third section the metabolic aspects; and the fourth section the physical body.

When a patient attends for treatment, they are asked to write their signature on the back of the chart, along the spine. Their signature contains their vibration and acts as a 'witness'. From this 'witness', the practitioner is able to dowse the spine in order to establish which of the vertebrae transmit a vibration. These 'active' vertebrae are marked and filled in with their correct colour. From these active vertebrae, the practitioner is able to discern what is happening to the patient on a mental, emotional, metabolic, and physical level.

On the chart, opposite the spine, are a line of thirty-two corresponding boxes. Into these are put the complementary colour to the marked and coloured vertebrae (see Fig. 11). A specific technique is then carried out from which the required colour and complementary colour can be established. This technique takes time to learn, but during the time I have used it I have found it to be very accurate and also a very useful tool in counselling.

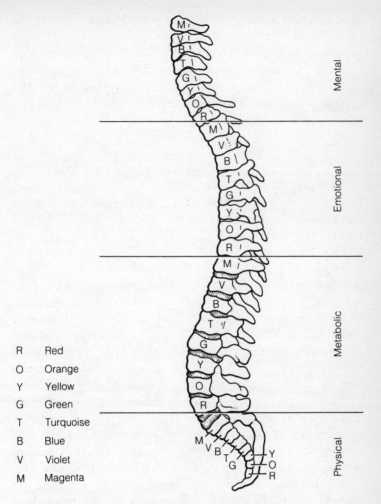

Fig. 10. The four sections of the spine

METHODS OF COLOUR TREATMENT

The Hygeia Colour Therapy Instrument

In order to treat a person with colour transmitted through stained glass filters, a colour therapy instrument has been devised by Theo Gimbel at the Hygeia College of Colour Therapy. This is approximately five feet in height, and comprises two large compartments, each of which is fitted

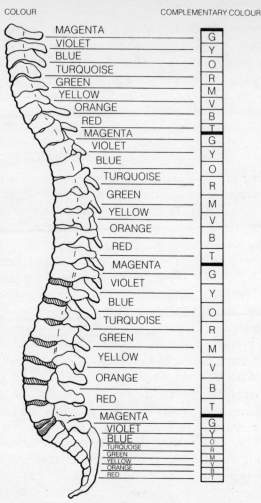

COLOUR   COMPLEMENTARY COLOUR

Fig. 11. Part of colour-diagnosis chart produced by the Hygeia College of Colour Therapy.

with a pure daylight bulb. The stained glass filter needed for the treatment colour, slides on to the front of the top section, and the complementary colour slides on to the front of the lower section. These two colours are then automatically administered to the patient in a rhythm which is based on the Fibonacci series of numbers in which each number is the sum of the previous two. In this rhythm, the treatment colour is initially given for a very short duration of time, while the complementary colour is given for a longer duration. During the course of the treatment this process is reversed, ending with a long exposure to the therapy colour and a short exposure to its complementary. When research was being carried out with this instrument, it was discovered that if the treatment colour and the complementary colour were each administered for periods of two minutes throughout the length of the treatment, after a short time the body 'switched off', no longer absorbing the colours transmitted. By basing the time changes of the colours on the Fibonacci series of numbers, a surprise element was introduced, and the colours continued to be absorbed by the patient, thus allowing the body to receive the maximum benefit from the therapy.

Masks are used with this colour therapy instrument. These are based upon the forms and complementary forms of the five platonic solids and are placed in front of the stained glass filters. The five platonic solids are the tetrahedron which has four faces and is related to the colour red; the octahedron which has eight faces and is related to the colour yellow; the hexahedron which has six faces and is related to the colour green; the icosahedron which has twenty faces and is related to the colour blue and the pentagondodechahedron which has twelve faces and is related to the colour violet. If we look into the cell structure of minerals, plants, animals and humans, we discover that they all follow the structure of the five platonic solids. Therefore, by using masks aligned with these structures, the whole treatment is improved. The total colour treatment lasts for just under twenty minutes (see Fig. 12).

This method is always given in a darkened room to prevent the colours from being diluted by daylight. The person receiving the treatment must be dressed completely in white so that there is no distortion of the colour being given. If someone is being treated with yellow light and they are wearing blue clothes, the colour which they receive will be a combination of the two, namely green.

Solarized Water

Stained glass filters can be used to solarize water or cream which is then administered to the patient in the dosage required.

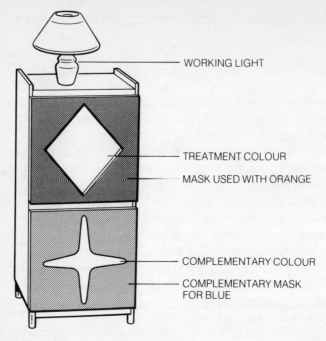

WORKING LIGHT

TREATMENT COLOUR

MASK USED WITH ORANGE

COMPLEMENTARY COLOUR

COMPLEMENTARY MASK
FOR BLUE

*Fig. 12. Diagram of colour therapy instrument produced by Hygeia
Studios*

To solarize water, one can either use stained glass bottles
or a water solarizer. Spring water is put into the bottles or
solarizer and left in the sun or strong daylight for several hours.
The theory behind this method is that, in passing through the
stained glass, the sun transmits the vibration of the colour into
the water. This method of treatment is being successfully used
by a medically qualified doctor and colour therapist in India.

During a summer school which I attended, a very interesting experiment was conducted by the students. Water
was put into eight different coloured solarizers and left in
the sun for the best part of the day. Towards evening,
each of the students was asked to taste the eight glasses
of colour-solarized water and to report their findings. Each
student independently noted that the eight glasses of water,
each solarized with a different colour, had a distinct taste.
Some were sweet, some sour, smooth, rough, and so on.
Note: when working with this, or any of the other methods
described, it is always advisable to seek the advice of a qualified

colour practitioner. (How to find a practitioner is given in a later chapter.)

Solarized Cream

Solarized cream works on the same principle. The cream must be pure, free from perfume, chemicals or preservatives. The ideal cream would be home made, although unfortunately this must be kept in a refrigerator, has a short life span, and does not take kindly to being left in the sun under stained glass. When a suitable cream has been selected, the desired amount is placed into a white container and the correct colour stained glass filter is placed over the top. This is then left in the sunlight for several hours. Solarized cream is used primarily for skin conditions.

Other Methods of Colour Treatment

Small stained glass filters can be used to concentrate colour on to a specific part of the body. For a finger infection, for example, a light can be shone through a turquoise filter which is held over the finger. For a cyst, a piece of green glass is used in the same way.

Another way of transmitting colour to a patient is by allowing it to be channelled through one's own physical body. One method of doing this is taught by the Maitreya School of Healing and is called 'Mental Colour Therapy'. A second method, taught by the Hygeia College of Colour Therapy, is called 'scanning'. The method which I use with most of my patients is derived from the teachings of both schools.

A COLOUR TREATMENT SESSION

Once it has been sensitized to colour, the physical body becomes a beautiful and accurate instrument. Through it colours can be channelled which as yet have not become manifest on earth.

There are many ways in which we can work to sensitize our body but it is important that we work at our own pace, allowing ourselves to unfold gently, like the petals of a flower.

I always teach my students to learn to feel colour through nature. The abundance and richness of nature's colours present a living energy, unlike the synthetic dyes used to colour man-made fibres. Next time you are in the country, by the sea or in the garden, be aware of the wonderful spectrum of colour which surrounds you. I am sure that your eyes will be opened to things that were previously unseen.

When working as a channel for colour healing, I have found it to be very important to dedicate myself to the Universal Spirit or God, and to ask that I may be a good channel in order to help the person I am about to treat.

After taking down the patient's particulars, medical history and current state of health, I make a colour diagnostic chart. This gives me insight into the mental, emotional, metabolic and physical state of the person, as well as providing the colour needed. This is followed by counselling and treatment.

For the treatment, the patient has the procedure explained to him/her and is then asked to lie on a therapy couch. They are then put into a state of relaxation. So many of today's illnesses are caused by stress, and to teach a person how to relax is a step towards helping them to help themselves. Also, tension in a patient can prevent them from receiving the full benefit of the treatment.

When the patient is relaxed and comfortable, the treatment starts with the technique known as 'scanning'. This entails sensing and feeling the aura through the hands. In the palm of each hand is a minor chakra or energy centre which, when open, act as eyes through which the therapist can see or feel energy blocks. When we discussed the aura, we learnt that it is here that dis-ease starts and if not eradicated manifests in the physical body. With this technique, knowledge can also be gained as to whether or not the chakras are functioning correctly. I have frequently found that due to emotional trauma or stress, these can be partially or completely blocked. When these blockages are detected, the therapist endeavours to clear them. This may not be possible in the first or second treatment; the longer the problem has been established, the longer it takes to clear.

After the aura has been scanned, and blockages worked with, the physical body is treated through touch. It is at this stage that colour is channelled through the therapist's hands and into the patient. Starting with the head, the therapist works down the body, gently touching it and visualizing the colours to be channelled. This can only be learnt through undertaking the necessary training. Sometimes the colour visualized will not be the colour which comes through. If one has dedicated oneself to be a channel for colour healing, one has to accept that God or the higher powers know better than we do and will channel through us the colour which is most beneficial for the patient.

The treatment ends by placing the palms of the hands on the soles of the patient's feet and visualizing gold energizing light streaming through their body. The therapist then asks that any negative or unwanted energies may be dispersed and that the auras of patient and therapist be separated. When one is working in this way, the auras of patient and therapist become intermingled, and if they are not separated at the end of treatment, it is possible for the therapist to remain in contact with the patient on a psychic level. This is not good for either.

The Colour Crystal Torch

With the above technique, a practitioner will sometimes use what is known as the 'Colour Crystal Torch'. This is a device in which light is shone through stained glass discs into a quartz crystal point (see Fig. 13).

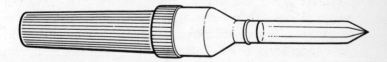

Fig. 13 Colour Crystal Torch

When this torch is used with the appropriate colour, it is able to balance the chakras or transmit colour to specific areas of the body. There is also a smaller version of the torch which is used in reflexology. When the torch is used, the patient must be dressed in white for the same reasons given when using the colour therapy instrument. I have white gowns which patients wear for this kind of treatment.

Use of Silks and the Colour Space Illuminator

When one treats with scanning, there are ways in which the therapy and complementary colour can be relayed to the patient during treatment.

The two methods which I use are: 1. by using lengths of pure silk material which have been dyed with natural dyes; and 2. with the aid of a lamp called the 'colour space illuminator'. This lamp can be tuned to flood the room with the desired colour. If the treatment colour needed is blue, the colour space illuminator is turned on to blue and floods the therapy room with this colour during treatment. When treatment is finished, the patient is left to rest for ten to fifteen minutes in the complementary colour, orange. Again, when using this lamp, the room has to be darkened to prevent the colour being diluted by the daylight.

If one is using silks, the patient is covered with the silk, corresponding to the treatment colour. This is then changed to the complementary coloured silk, after treatment. When using silks, the patient should be treated in a bright and, if possible, sunny room in order that the light transmits the maximum amount of colour into the patient as it passes through the silk.

It is also possible to use both the silks and the colour space illuminator during a treatment. Each practitioner determines what they use by what they feel will be most beneficial for the patient.

AURA SOMA

This is a completely different form of colour therapy from those already mentioned. It was the invention of Vicky Wall, a pharmacist and chiropodist. When she went blind, her 'inner' sight developed, enabling her to see people's auras clearly.

Aura Soma combines aspects of herbal medicine, aromatherapy and mineral supplementation with colour therapy. It consists of pairs of coloured oils, forming an upper and lower layer within a set of bottles. Vicky Wall referred to these as 'balances'. When a patient came for treatment, she would ask them to choose a bottle, believing that the colour they chose related to their own energy field and that their attraction to certain colours meant that they needed its reinforcing power. She would then ask the patient to shake the bottle. From the turbulence created in the oils, she was able to read the state of the patient's energy field. She believed that in healthy people, the oils quickly regained their respective layers, while in unhealthy people, a cloudy effect was produced which took time to clear.

To discover which parts of a patient's body lacked harmony, she herself would shake the chosen bottle at specific points in the patient's aura. According to whether the oils went cloudy or stayed opaque she knew if there was disease in the corresponding part of the physical body. At the end of treatment, the patient was instructed to take the chosen bottle home and to look at it daily in order to absorb its vital energy.

These oils that she created can be used as massage or bath oils. Using the oils in either of these ways again allows their vital energy to be absorbed into the physical body.

Sadly for us, Vicky Wall is now in spirit, but Aura Soma lives on. Details of their venue can be found at the end of this book.

REFLEXOLOGY AND COLOUR

Colour can also be used in conjunction with other therapies. I use it with both reflexology and yoga.

Being both a qualified reflexologist and colour practitioner enabled me to do two years' research into the effects of combining both these therapies. To begin with I would carry out a normal reflexology treatment, this being very valuable both as a therapy and also as a diagnostic tool. After this I applied colour to the reflexes which were painful and those which related to the problem which had caused the patient to seek help. In cases where the feet were too painful to touch, I treated with colour alone. The results were truly amazing. This encouraged me to run courses for reflexologists who wished to use colour to support the therapy which they were already practising. I asked those who attended the courses to report their findings to me. They were all favourable and we realized that colour used in this way treated a patient on all three aspects of their being; body, mind and spirit. One reflexologist reported that one of her patients had told her that colour reaches the parts that a therapist cannot! For further information read my book *The Reflexology and Colour Therapy Workbook* published by Element Books.

YOGA AND COLOUR

Having taught and practised yoga for many years, I quickly realized that apart from being a discipline and a path in life, it could also be categorized as a holistic therapy. When working with *asanas* (postures), one also works with the chakras, which in turn affect the endocrine glands. As already explained, each chakra radiates a dominant colour. Knowing this and knowing the important part that the ductless glands play in the harmonization of the physical body, I introduced to my students the idea of visualizing the appropriate chakra and its dominant colour whilst holding a posture. From this we worked with colour in breathing, visualization and meditation. I found this to be an exciting venture with beneficial results. A deeper insight into this can be obtained through reading *Sixteen Steps to Health and Energy* which I co-wrote with Theo. Gimbel and which is published by Quantum.

GEM STONES

The techniques for transmitting colour contained in this chapter, are ones which I have personally experienced or worked with. There are many more, such as the use of gem stones. Each stone resonates to its own sound and is illuminated with its chosen colour. When used in healing, these stones are laid in precise patterns on the physical body. They can also be used to align and balance the chakras. In order to do this, the correct coloured gem is placed on each of the seven chakras. For example, lapis lazuli or sapphire is placed on the throat chakra, both vibrating to the blue ray.

If one does not have the correct coloured gems, it is possible to solarize quartz crystal. A piece of quartz is placed on to a lamp, which is fitted with the correct stained glass filter and left for thirty to sixty minutes. If this technique is used, the crystal must be cleansed after use by placing it in salt water for twelve hours or by leaving it in a free-flowing brook. All gems that are used in therapy should be cleansed in this way after each treatment.

If you wish to know more about gem therapy, there are many excellent books on the market written by people who are both experienced and qualified in this field.

CONCLUSION

When a patient attends for treatment, they are always advised of ways in which they can help themselves with colour. If we stop and look around us and also take note of the colours of the clothes which we are wearing, we will realize that we are, in small potencies, continually being treated with colour.

Having said this, may I close this chapter by saying that if you have a problem, it is always advisable to seek the advice and help of a colour practitioner rather than try to treat yourself.

5

What Colour Can Do For You

COLOUR IS A holistic treatment, working with a person on the spiritual, mental, emotional and physical levels. It treats the whole person, not just the disease. Because of this, it can help all who choose to be treated by it, including animals and plants.

Animals and plants respond beautifully to colour treatment for they erect no barriers through not fully understanding or believing its curative powers. They just accept.

I have a wonderful cat called Suzie. She became ill with a high temperature and refused to eat or drink. She just lay listless on a chair. I took her to the vet and he said that she had picked up a virus. He gave her an antibiotic injection and prescribed antibiotic tablets. The tablets had an adverse effect and she got worse instead of better. In desperation, I treated her with colour by allowing it to be channelled through me. She lay very still whilst I placed my hands over her body. Two hours after treatment, she started to lap water. I carried her and put her on to my bed, this being where she normally sleeps, and gave her another treatment before I went to sleep. In the middle of the night, I was woken by a furry head and purring body trying to get into bed with me. The next morning she ate a little food. I gave her two further treatments and she made an exceedingly fast recovery.

If we, as humans, could completely accept in the same way as animals do, then colour would work wonders for us. Unfortunately, we are endowed with a thinking capacity which enables us to intellectualize and to erect barriers. It is these which stop us responding. This has been proven in the use of placebos. Patients, some of whom have been terminally ill, have been given placebos, believing them to be a new drug which is capable of curing their disease. Believing this, they have actually started to recover. When they find out that the supposedly new drug is in fact only a tablet composed of sugar and water, they immediately go into relapse. This shows how the mind affects the body. In the same way, the body can affect the mind. There are times when it is to our advantage to adopt the trust of a child or animal.

When a person attends for treatment, they are always asked if they have sought the advice of their doctor. If not, they are recommended to do so. I feel very strongly that complementary medicine should be what its name implies. Complementary to orthodox medicine. If they choose not to seek medical advice, then that is their choice and responsibility.

If a patient has undergone surgery, then colour therapy can speed their recovery. If they are receiving treatment for a disease, whether of long or short duration, colour can again assist with this.

CASE HISTORIES

Physical Conditions

Mr. A had just come home from hospital, having undergone a heart by-pass operation the previous week. His wife came to me and asked if I could help him. She said that he was depressed and anxious, and was experiencing a great deal of tension around his neck and shoulders as well as pain in his chest where his rib cage has been opened in order to gain access to the heart. I said that I would try and arranged to visit him.

I found Mr. A to be a very sensitive and gentle man, but unable to talk about his own feelings. He said that he had always had this problem. He confirmed what his wife had already told me – that he was unable to sleep due to the pain in his shoulders, neck and chest. I carried out a colour treatment, finishing by massaging his neck and shoulders with solarized oil. I recommended that he take arnica tablets, a homeopathic remedy for shock and bruising, and arranged to give him another treatment in three days' time. The next day, his wife telephoned to say that he had slept soundly and that he had made a marked improvement.

On the next visit, he said that he felt much better but was still having neck and shoulder pains. After the normal colour treatment, I again massaged his neck and shoulders with solarized oil. He said that this gave him great relief and was very relaxing. When I attended him a week later, he looked much better. Treatment was continued at weekly intervals for a further six weeks, by the end of which time he had made a complete recovery.

Colour practitioners never claim to cure people. The only person who can bring about a cure is the person to whom the ailment belongs. For this to happen, the cause must be found and worked with. For many people, this can be a very painful procedure.

Counselling plays a very important part in colour therapy. Colour practitioners frequently find that those attending for help have no one in whom they can confide. Because the practitioner is a stranger, and because they are under no obligation to see her/him again, they feel that they can pour out their hearts, and thus experience tremendous relief.

I always tell patients that whatever they say never finds its way outside the therapy room, and that once they have left I have the ability to forget what they have said, only remembering it on their next visit. May I say, that it is vital for practitioners to acquire this technique, for if they do not they could find themselves carrying around all of their patients' unwanted baggage as well as their own.

Mrs F attended with a broken wrist which had happened through falling whilst out shopping. She had been taken to hospital where her arm and hand were x-rayed prior to being put into a plaster cast. Her main complaint was of pain. She had been prescribed painkillers but found that they made her feel unwell. A full colour treatment was given, with emphasis on the arm and broken wrist. After treatment, she said that she felt the pain diminishing when colour was being channelled through her wrist. During the following week, I gave her two further treatments, both of which greatly reduced the pain.

When she next attended hospital, they were delighted with her progress and were able to remove the plaster sooner than expected. She was delighted, but confessed that she did not have the courage to tell the hospital staff that she had been treated with colour!

Mrs. G attended with rheumatoid arthritis, a disease characterized by inflammation of joints, swelling, pain, and loss of function. The onset of this had been several years previously and had started after a fall. She had been treated with anti-inflammatory drugs and for a short time had been given steroids. Because of the side effects, she had asked to be taken off these. The main joints affected were her fingers, wrists and neck. We talked about diet, hers not being very satisfactory, and agreed that she should make an appointment with a dietician. This she did. During treatment, special attention was paid to the inflamed joints. After treatment, these were massaged with solarized oil and she was instructed to do the same. She attended for treatment on a weekly basis for a period of four months. This, combined with her new diet, produced a marked improvement. The last time I saw her, her joints were still a little stiff, but the swelling and pain had been eradicated.

Mr. H attended with chronic sinus problems which had been with him for many years. He had sought medical advice but never followed the treatment prescribed. He was one of life's real characters – always laughing and joking and, to put it mildly, a little overweight. I asked him why he wanted to be treated with colour. His reply was that he had heard about it from his mate who had read about it in a magazine and he was game to try anything. I questioned him on diet and it transpired that he ate large quantities of dairy produce. I advised him to give this up because it could be irritating his existing condition. With a twinkle in his eye, he promised me that he would try. He continued to have treatment on a weekly basis for a month, and on each of these visits I enquired about his intake of dairy produce. With the same twinkle in his eye and smile on his face, he informed me that he hadn't quite got round to not eating it but intended to do so. On his last visit, he was still eating vast amounts of dairy produce and his sinuses were still as bad. I looked at him in despair. With a broad grin and a chuckle, he told me that he had loved the experience of colour and would not have missed it for the world. Regarding his intake of dairy produce? He was still thinking about it! I wonder if he will ever eliminate it from his diet. Somehow, I doubt it!

Unfortunately, a lot of people seek colour therapy as a last resort, having been told that nothing else can be done for them. This usually means that by the time they are seen by a complementary practitioner, the disease from which they are suffering is so far advanced that the only help that can be given is relief from pain with love. I personally believe that there are people who, when they reincarnate into a physical body, choose to experience death through a particular disease. When this happens, the task of the practitioner is to help them through the transition with love and counselling.

I believe Miss J was one such person. She was young and attended with advanced breast cancer. One breast was an open, ulcerated wound, where the tumour had broken through the skin, and the other breast was solid with tumour which was also on the verge of breaking the skin. Miss J was a very bright and cheerful person. She had great faith in complementary therapy and had been treated with this since the discovery of the initial breast lump. I first saw her about three months before she died, and during these months she came regularly for treatment. This relieved most of the pain that she was experiencing. We talked a great deal about the process of death and life after death, which she firmly believed in. I never once heard her complain or found her despondent, and she never gave up hope of being cured. When she died, she was at home with her family, was very peaceful and free from pain.

A question which I am often asked by my patients is: 'Will I feel anything during treatment?' The answer is that some people do and others do not. What is and what is not felt depends upon the sensitivity of the recipient. Normally I do not encourage patients to talk during treatment, the main reasons for this being, firstly, that it prevents them from relaxing, and, secondly, that it interferes with my concentration. There was however one exception to this rule.

Mrs. J attended with menopausal problems. Believing the menopause to be a natural process, she did not wish to take hormone replacement therapy. We talked about this, and my belief that during the menopause, the earthly energies which were used in childbearing are changed into spiritual energies. In many of the ancient teachings, this was the time when a woman became a priestess or goddess. So many woman today think that once they reach this stage in their life they are getting old and that life is no longer worth living. Many of them try to regain their youth and beauty, sometimes by going to the extreme of having cosmetic surgery. If only they realized that beauty comes from within! Yes, the menopause is a time of change, a change into the next stage of life. If looked at in the correct way, it can be exciting, rewarding and adventurous. I agree that some menopausal symptoms are unpleasant, but most changes, in whatever form they occur, bring some discomfort.

After conversing on this for some time, I gave Mrs. J treatment, firstly putting her into relaxation and then scanning her aura. When I came to work with her chakras, she started telling me the colours which she was seeing behind closed eyes. I found this fascinating. Sometimes they were the same colour as I was visualizing and sometimes not. I must admit that on this occasion I worked for a longer period of time on her chakras than I normally would.

When I had completed her treatment, we talked about her experiences. She admitted that she was very sensitive to colour in her surroundings and in the clothes which she wore. She experienced the same phenomenon during subsequent treatments.

Some patients 'feel' rather than 'see' the colour which is being channelled. Some experience what they describe as energy flowing through their body. Others experience heat and/or a prickling sensation on the area of their body being treated. I have had patients involuntarily move their limbs, head or torso. When they ask what is happening, I have to explain that I do not know, that I am just a channel and whatever happens during treatment is to the benefit of the patient.

There have been occasions when patients have reported 'other' people besides myself touching them. I tell them that these are my unseen helpers in the spirit world who work with me.

Mental/Emotional Conditions

Some months ago, a Mr B came to me for treatment. He complained of palpitations and anxiety attacks. He had attended his doctor who had confirmed that there was no heart problem, and prescribed tranquillizers. During our conversation, I detected that all was not well with his home life. I casually asked him about this and he assured me that his home life was wonderful. On his second visit, I made a colour diagnostic chart and this confirmed what I had detected. I went through the chart with him explaining that it showed emotional trauma which was being released by his physical body through the symptoms that he was experiencing. Again he reassured me that all was well; that he had a wonderful wife and family. On his third visit, I again broached the subject of his wife and family. This was followed by silence which lasted for almost fifteen minutes after which he began to talk and talk, pouring out all of his problems, especially the problem of his relationship with his wife. He confessed that he had never been able to speak about this to anyone else and I believe that he felt embarrassed that he had confided in me. After this, I did not see him again for treatment for about three weeks. He reported that he felt much better and, with the permission of his doctor, had stopped taking tranquillizers. He said that he had as yet been unable to find a solution to his problem, but the fact that he had been able to verbalize it and acknowledge its presence had brought him halfway to solving it and curing himself.

Another patient, Mrs. C, came complaining of depression and lack of energy. She herself was a complementary practitioner and felt that she was not a good example to her patients. Because of this, she was not seeing any new patients and was gradually letting her practice close down. We talked about her work and her family, about which she was very non-committal, before I made a colour diagnostic chart.

The chart showed that there was a great deal of emotional and mental trauma and hardly any joy in her life. She then told me that her marriage was deteriorating and through her husband failing to love and understand her she had found someone else. This went against her moral principles and what she really wanted was for her husband to provide what the other man was giving her. We talked about the various avenues which she could take before I gave her treatment. On her second visit, she said that she had thought about everything we had discussed and had decided that she wanted to tell her husband the truth. The next time I heard from her was by letter. She had told her husband the truth. Initially he was very angry and upset, but they had eventually talked and were both working to establish a greater understanding of each other.

Some patients find it almost impossible to talk about themselves and their problems. Anger and frustration is bottled up inside them literally eating them away. If nothing is done, this state can result in cancer.

I have found with this type of person that treating them with colour can actually help them to talk. In my experience, the colour breaks down long-established barriers, rather like removing dams which have been built to stop the flow of water. Once the dam has been removed, they start to cry and this relieves their inner tension.

Mr D came to see me complaining of digestive disorders. He had attended his doctor and undergone various tests to try and locate the problem. He came from India and was a Hindu. On a recent visit to India, he had undertaken various holistic therapies which had given him some relief. He explained that on the last visit he had undergone an arranged marriage but had had to return without his bride because of immigration problems. He was at present living with his parents. He said that his only problem was his inability to work full time due to his sickness. I made a colour diagnostic chart for him and carried out treatment.

On his second visit, he said that he had experienced slight relief for a few days but then the digestive problem had reverted to its previous state. I tried to encourage him to talk about himself, but he felt that there was very little to say. When I started to treat and channel colour into his solar plexus, I felt as though my hands were being held there for much longer then is normal. I then became aware that Mr D was desperately fighting to stop himself crying. I removed my hands from his solar plexus and held his hands, encouraging him to cry. Eventually he did, after which he started to talk.

His problem was a very difficult one. Basically, he did not wish to be married. He was the eldest son and this, in his culture, made him responsible for his younger brothers and sister. He felt that this responsibility was more than he could handle. On top of this, he had been under obligation to go through with his arranged marriage which burdened him with more responsibility. His way of solving the problem was to become ill. If he was ill, he would not be expected to shoulder the responsibilities which had been placed upon him. The colour treatment and finally being able to talk freely helped him to look at and work with himself. By doing this, he was gradually able to start to undertake his responsibilities.

Mrs E came to me complaining of depression and a weight problem. She told me that she lived alone, was at present unemployed due to ill health, but wanted to train as a complementary practitioner. We talked about this and her health problems. Her colour diagnostic chart showed joylessness, emotional trauma, disturbance in the digestive system, and lack of physical energy. When I explained this to her, she confessed that she was suffering from bulimia, a disorder characterized by overeating, followed by self-induced vomiting. This usually occurs in response to fears of being overweight, stress and depression. I asked if she had sought medical help. She replied that she had not and had no wish to do so. When I treated her with colour, I felt that she was trying to resist. When we discussed this, she agreed but did not know the reason why. On her second visit, I again felt this resistance during treatment. I quietly tuned into my own intuition, asking what to do. I was guided to work on her heart chakra, and this I did. Gradually the resistance started to break down and she began to cry. I held her head, and after she had quietened down, she started to talk.

She told me that she had been unloved as a child and had always sought love which she then found difficult to accept. When she left school she worked in catering, gradually climbing the ladder to the point where she was running a well-established and flourishing restaurant. She worked very hard, having very little time for herself. During this period in her life, she became involved in a relationship with one of the staff, who hurt her very badly, finally walking out on her for someone else. The outcome for her, was a nervous breakdown. She had to give up work and sought comfort in eating.

I worked with her over a three-month period, during which time she gradually started to heal. She made enquiries into and attended workshops on a variety of complementary therapies, and she also found herself a part-time job. The last time I saw her, she had started to lose weight and was working very hard with herself. She still had the occasional relapse, but these were getting fewer.

ABSENT HEALING

For many reasons, some people are unable to attend the place where I work and write requesting absent healing Frequently the request is for a friend or loved one. In this situation, I always ask that they obtain the permission of the person for whom they are requesting healing. Absent healing can activate changes in the person being treated and if they are not aware that they are receiving healing these changes could cause them concern. I also feel that it is an infringement on a person's free will to work on them without their permission.

In order to treat a patient from a distance, a witness, in the form of a photograph, a lock of hair or their handwriting is required. This is placed underneath the diagnostic spine chart prior to dowsing and compiling it. Once the chart has been made, this in itself being a form of treatment, absent healing can be carried out in two ways:

The first is by administering the correct colours, through the colour crystal torch, to the 'active' vertebrae shown on the spine chart. Each active vertebra receives approximately a fifteen-second treatment. This is only carried out once on each individual spine chart.

The second method is through visualization. The patient is visualized lying either on a therapy couch or in a beautiful garden. The colours which they require are then mentally projected to the appropriate parts of their body. As these colours are received, the patient is visualized as becoming

81

well and strong with all disease eradicated. The treatment ends by enfolding them in an orb of golden light for energy and protection.

With both of these methods a written report on the spine chart is made and sent to the patient. In this report advice is given on self-help with colour, and on diet if this is relevant.

A short time ago, I received a request by post for absent healing. This request had come from a former patient for her husband. The only information she gave me was that he was suffering from severe depression. I wrote back, enclosing a spine chart for her husband to sign and requesting that she told him about the treatment.

The spine chart was returned a few days later. She confirmed that she had explained this and the healing procedure to her husband. Apparently he was very sceptical but had signed the chart in order to please his wife.

When the chart was completed it showed a lack of emotional, mental and physical joy, thus causing a state of lethargy. The mental aspect of the chart revealed a turbulent state of mind. He was obviously very anxious about something which he felt unable to talk about, and this was causing him to feel a lack of self-respect and dignity.

I sent his wife a report on my findings. A week later, I received a letter from her telling me that she had imparted the information to her husband, after which he had remained silent for some time. He had then broken down and told her that he was on the point of being made redundant. This had worried him a great deal, causing loss of sleep and a feeling of no longer being useful to society. He had kept this information to himself in order not to worry his wife.

After they had been able to talk and discuss all the possible avenues which were open to him, he told her that he felt as though a tremendous weight had been lifted. She was equally delighted that he had confided in her, making it possible for them to share and tackle the problem together.

Throughout the years that I have been working with colour, I have seen the many wonderful ways in which it has helped people. Some readers may find this difficult to believe, and if this is the case, may I suggest that you experience the therapeutic power of colour for yourself, by visiting a colour practitioner.

6

How to Help Yourself with Colour

I F YOU ARE ILL, whether with a major or minor problem, or if
you are under stress or generally feeling tired and lethargic,
there are many ways in which you can help yourself with colour. I must, however, stress again the importance of initially
seeking the advice of a qualified colour practitioner who will be
able to advise you on the best method of self help. If something
has gone wrong with your physical body, it can indicate that
a change in life style is needed. For many people this can be
very difficult. The simple self help measures outlined in this
chapter can be used by anyone.

One of the major causes of disease in our present age is stress.
As we enter the Aquarian age, planet earth and its inhabitants
are undergoing many changes. Many people are finding their
life style, relationships and patterns of life being broken down
in order that new ones may be established. This can lead to a
sense of insecurity and bewilderment. Frequently it leaves us
with a feeling of aloneness, of not knowing where the next
step will lead, and sometimes not knowing in which direction
the next step should be taken. For us to evolve on to a higher
level of spiritual awareness, change has to take place. If we are
unable to accept this and to flow with the tide of life, then we
create anxiety and stress within ourselves. This prevents our
physical body from functioning to its full potential and will
eventually lead to disease. If we are aware that we are under
stress, then we can use colour to help release it. The colour
normally used for this is blue.

For this exercise, you will need a full length piece of blue silk or cotton. Making sure that you are dressed in white, lie down in a warm, sunny or well-lit room. Make sure that your body is straight, feet slightly apart and the palms of your hands facing toward the ceiling. Place a pillow under your head to prevent any strain on the cervical spine. If you find it helpful, have music quietly playing in the room. Cover your body with the length of blue silk. Try to relax your mind, letting go of any thoughts. Visualize these as beautiful bubbles which float into the atmosphere and gently disperse as you let go of them. When you have quietened your mind, focus it on your physical body. Starting at your toes and slowly working towards your head, try to release any tension, allowing your body to become heavy and relaxed. When you have completed this, rest your mind in the music, allowing the blue rays to be absorbed into your body. This exercise can be practised twice daily.

Different coloured silks can be used for specific ailments – for example, yellow for arthritic conditions, and orange for depression. The only exceptions to this are red and green which should only be used under the guidance of a colour practitioner.

YOGA EXERCISES WITH COLOUR VISUALIZATION

Another way of releasing stress is through exercise. The pace of modern life leaves many of us with very little time to exercise our bodies. People frequently tell me that they have ample exercise during normal working hours, achieved by walking to the bus stop or station, climbing stairs shopping and walking from office to office, from department to department. What they fail to realize is that this form of exercise is normally carried out under stress, their mind being occupied with the many tasks waiting to be completed. True exercise releases stress. This is only possible if the mind is relaxed and able to concentrate on what the body is doing.

There are many excellent forms of exercise which remove stress and relax the body. One which I have worked with for many years is the discipline of yoga, which can be used very effectively in conjunction with colour.

Each posture, or asana, works with one of the main chakras and its associated endocrine gland. When practising asanas, it is the length of time the posture is held that matters – not the number of repetitions. A beginner to yoga will hold each posture for a relatively short time, the time being gradually increased as the body becomes stronger and more supple. It is during the holding of a posture that one firstly learns to visualize and become aware of its associated chakra and then to visualize the colour which radiates from it. By working with all seven chakras during a practice session, all the seven colours are equally brought into play, thereby releasing stress, re-energizing the body and bringing it back into harmony.

Yoga is a discipline, a way of life, and anyone wishing to study this art seriously should do so under the guidance of an experienced teacher. To learn it initially from books is not advisable, for in order to gain maximum benefit from a posture, the body must be positioned correctly, and this is difficult to ascertain without the guidance of an instructor. When working with *pranayama* (breathing techniques) and meditation, both of which are part of yoga, certain rules apply. If not applied correctly, you could do yourself harm instead of good.

Seven simple postures are shown below, each of which activates one of the chakras. When working with these, please practise all seven in every session. Dress in loose, comfortable clothing, and allow four hours to elapse since your last meal. If possible try to practise at the same time each day as this creates a discipline which will help you to practise regularly. The ideal time is in the morning as soon as you have risen from bed, but unfortunately this is the time when the body is stiff and least flexible. Do not worry if you cannot manage the full posture. Be aware of your body and do not strain. When you have reached your maximum position in each of the postures, hold it, and try to visualize the relevant colour radiating from the chakra into your aura. You will find the position of the chakras depicted in Fig. 9 on p. 46.

Before starting your session, lie down and relax your body for five to ten minutes. It is much easier to move a relaxed body than one that is tense. Do likewise at the end of each session.

Red – Muladhara or Base Chakra

The Knee Lock

Lie on the floor, on your back, with your legs together and your hands by your sides. Tuck your chin into your chest in order to extend the cervical spine. Breathe in and bend your right knee up to your chest, clasping it with both hands. Make sure that your left leg remains in a relaxed position on the floor. Breathe out and bring your head as near as possible to your knee. Using a shallow breath, hold the posture for as long as is comfortable while bringing your concentration into the base chakra. Visualize the beautiful clear colour of red radiating from this chakra and flowing into your aura. Breathe in and lie back on to the floor. Repeat with your left leg and then work both legs together.

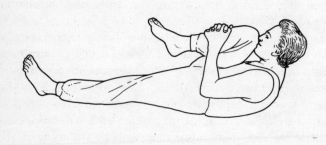

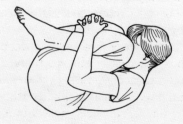

Fig. 14. The Knee Lock

Orange – Swadisthana or Sacral Centre

Padangusthasana – Hand to Foot Posture

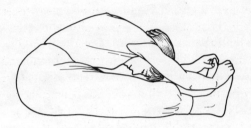

Fig. 15. Hand to Foot Posture

Stand on the floor with your feet approximately fifteen centimetres apart. Make sure that your feet are parallel with the toes of your left and right feet in line with each. Straighten your spine by imagining that you have a balloon attached to the crown of your head, which is gently lifting up your body. On your next outbreath, bend the trunk of your body forward from the hips and hold your big toes with your hands. Hold this position and breathe in. On your next exhalation, keeping your spine straight, knees locked and without strain, continue to lower your trunk on to your legs. When you have reached your maximum posture, focus your attention on the sacral chakra, visualizing a clear bright orange streaming from it and radiating out into your aura. Hold for as long as is comfortable before inhaling and returning to the standing posture. *Caution* – Not to be practised by people with back ailments or sciatica. *Benefits* – This posture removes excess fat and eliminates flatulence, constipation and indigestion. It makes the spine and back muscles supple. All the spinal nerves are stimulated and toned and the metabolism is increased. It influences the reproductive system, removing sexual ailments. It gives a good flow of blood to the face and brain.

Yellow – The Manipura or Solar Plexus Chakra

Ustrasana – The Camel

Kneel on the floor with your feet and knees together and your toes tucked under. Place your right hand on your right heel and your left hand on your left heel. Press your hands down on to your feet. Carefully take your head back, and arch your spine until your thighs are in line with your knees. While you are holding this posture, bring your concentration into your solar plexus. Visualize a beautiful, clear yellow radiating from this chakra and expanding into your aura. When you get tired, release your hands, sit back on your legs and relax.

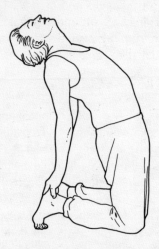

Fig. 16. The Camel

Benefits – This posture stretches and tones the whole of the spine, making it supple. It also works on the abdominal organs and muscles and on the shoulder joints.

Green – Anahata or Heart Chakra

The Warrior

Stand with your feet together, spine straight and shoulders back, in order to open your chest. Breathe in and jump your feet one metre apart. (If you suffer with back problems, 'walk' your feet apart). Turn your right foot outwards to 90°, and your left foot slightly in to the right. Breathing out, bend your right knee to form a right angle. This should bring your knee into line with your ankle. Stretch out your arms horizontally and turn your head to look at your right hand. Feel as though each of your hands is being held and pulled in order to open and expand your chest. Concentrate on your heart centre, visualizing a clear bright green radiating from it and flowing into your aura, enabling your energies to be brought into balance. When your body tires, breathe in and return to the standing posture. Relax for a few seconds before repeating on the other side.

Caution – Should not be done by people with a weak heart.
Benefits – This posture opens and expands the chest allowing for deeper breathing. It strengthens the leg muscles and relieves cramp in the calf and thigh muscles. This posture helps to strengthen the entire body.

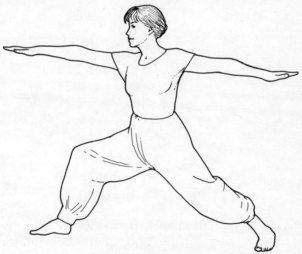

Fig. 17. The Warrior

Blue – *Visshuddhi or Throat Centre*

Ardha Chandrasana – The Crescent Moon

Kneel on the floor with your legs together and your arms by your sides. Bring the sole of your right foot on to the floor, making a right angle with your knee. Breathing in, stretch your left leg backwards, placing the palms of your hands on the floor on either side of your right foot. Breathe in. On your next outbreath, continue to move the left leg backwards, at the same time arching your back and taking your head back. Allow your hands to come off the floor until just your fingertips are touching. Hold this position and visualize a clear blue radiating from your throat chakra and into your aura. When you get tired, return to the kneeling position, relax for a minute and then repeat on the other side. *Benefits* – This posture strengthens and makes supple the whole of the skeletal structure.

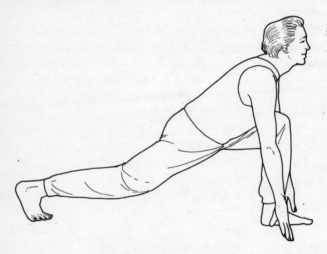

Fig. 18. The Crescent Moon

Indigo – Ajna or Brow Centre

Ardha Matsyendrasana – Half Abdominal Twist (Simple Version)

Sit on the floor with your legs stretched out in front of you. Bend your left knee, taking the left leg over the right leg and placing the sole of the left foot on the floor next to the right knee. Turn the trunk of your body towards the left leg. Bend the right elbow in front of your left knee. Take the left arm back, placing the palm of the hand on the floor behind the body, with the fingers pointing away from the body. Press the right arm and left knee against each other, rotating the trunk of the body as far to the left as possible. Look over your left shoulder and hold for as long as is comfortable. Whilst holding, bring your concentration into the brow centre, visualizing a deep indigo radiating from this centre and flowing out into your aura. When you are ready, repeat on the other side. *Caution* – Should not be done in the later stages of pregnancy. *Benefits* – This posture makes the spine and back muscles supple, helping to eliminate lumbago and muscular rheumatism. Because this posture works on the spine, it also works on the spinal nerves. It massages the abdominal organs and removes digestive ailments. It tones the kidneys, adrenal glands and pancreas. It is therefore a good posture for people suffering from diabetes.

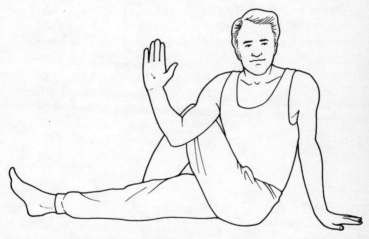

Fig. 19. Half Abdominal Twist

Violet – Sahasrara or Crown Centre

Prasarita Padottanasana – The Expanded Foot Posture

Stand on the floor with your feet together, spine straight, shoulders back and chest expanded. Breathing in, either jump or walk your feet approximately one metre apart. Make sure that your feet are parallel to each other and your toes in line. Breathing out and keeping your spine straight, extend the trunk of your body forward from the hips, placing the palms of your hands on the floor, with your fingers facing forward. If your body is stiff, preventing your hands from reaching the floor, use a wooden brick or books to place your hands on. This is the intermediate posture. If you have been able to place your hands on to the floor, slowly walk them backwards until they are in line with your feet. At the same time, extend your spine until the top of your head rests on the floor between your hands. When you have reached your maximum position, bring your awareness into the top of your head, visualizing a clear bright violet radiating from your crown chakra and flowing into your aura. As soon as you start to feel tired, come back to the standing posture and walk your feet together. *Caution –* People with high blood pressure should not hold this posture more than sixty seconds. *Benefits –* This posture works on the inner thighs and hamstring muscles. It removes stiffness from the shoulders and fully opens the chest. A fresh supply of blood flows to the head, neck and trunk of the body. This posture can be done by people who are unable to do the full head balance.

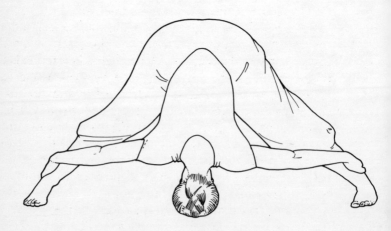

Fig. 20. The Expanded Foot Posture

When you have completed the seven postures and are lying on the floor with your body completely relaxed, try to become aware of any changes which may have taken place, physically, mentally or emotionally. You may not become aware of any changes until you have been practising regularly for several weeks, so do not be disappointed and give up if initially you feel that you are not benefiting from the practice of these postures.

CONTEMPLATION USING COLOUR

Another way of helping yourself with colour is through contemplation. This is an excellent method for relaxing both body and mind. Anything from nature can be used: flowers, stones, crystals, leaves, fruit, to name but a few. Each time that you work with this method, try to select a different colour and object.

Pink Rose Contemplation

For the following exercise you will need a pink rose, pink being the colour of unconditional love.

Take your rose and put it into a vase of water. Sit in a comfortable position, with the vase containing the rose at face level and about two feet away from you.

Relax your body and mind, bringing your concentration to the rose. Notice how it is formed; how the petals are attached to the stem; the delicacy of each petal and their individuality; the variation of the colour depicted by shadow and light. When you have gleaned as much visual information as you can, take the rose and lay it on the palm of your left hand. Place the palm of your right hand approximately two inches above the rose. Close your eyes and try to feel the vibration of the rose through your hands. If you feel nothing, do not be disappointed. It takes time and practice to sensitize the body to colour.

Place the rose back into the vase and, sitting quietly with your eyes closed, visualize the pink exhibited by the rose entering your heart chakra with each inhalation. On each exhalation, allow the colour to flow into your aura until you are sitting in an orb of pale pink light and are filled with spiritual, unconditional love. When you feel ready, resume normal breathing and gently open your eyes. Pale pink is one of the colours used for people who are experiencing emotional trauma.

Visualizing and breathing in colour is an excellent way of introducing colour into the body, and can be used for many of the conditions and states relating to the physical body. If you have difficulty in visualizing colour, find the colour you require in nature and closely study it prior to breathing it in.

Insomnia Exercise

Breathing in colour is a wonderful way of working with insomnia from which so many people suffer. In desperation, people will often resort to sleeping pills, but over a period of time the body gets used to these and they become less effective. When and if they are stopped, it takes time for the body to return to its natural rhythm, and once again, many sleepless nights are experienced.

If you suffer from insomnia, try the following exercise. Firstly, make sure that your body is comfortable and warm. Mentally go over your body, releasing any tension. After you have done this, visualize a beautiful deep blue, and on each inhalation, take this colour into your body. Feel it encompassing every muscle, organ and cell. If it helps, you can imagine your body to be a very special container which you are slowly filling with blue light. Continue to do this until you drift into sleep. Do not be disappointed and give up if your initial attempts fail. All that is needed is patient practice.

If you suffer from insomnia, you might also try sleeping in a blue nightdress between blue sheets. Having a low wattage blue light burning during the night will also help. It is only by trying these suggestions that you will discover the method best suited to you.

Exercise for Depression

Colour breathing can be used for depression. If you are suffering from this, sit down during the course of the day and follow the above method, breathing in orange instead of blue. It is not advisable to work with orange late at night because it is one of the energizing colours and could interfere with sleep.

Exercise for Arthritis

For arthritis, sit down, relax your body and breathe in yellow. Visualize this colour saturating the joints which are affected. From my own experience, I have found that diet also plays a crucial role in this sometimes crippling disease.

Energizing Exercise

To energize and bring the whole of the body back into balance, all of the colours are used in conjunction with the chakras:

Lie down in a comfortable position, making sure that your body is warm. Starting with your feet and working up through your body to your head, systematically relax each part. When you have done this, bring your concentration to your breathing. Feel the breath entering your nostrils and passing down into your lungs. Be aware of your chest expanding as your lungs inflate. Breathing out, feel the warm air passing out of your nostrils as your chest contracts with the deflation of your lungs.

Visualize a bright red rose. On your next inhalation, breathe this colour in through the soles of your feet and into the base chakra. As you exhale, watch this red colour radiating out from the base chakra, into your aura. The inhalation and exhalation is carried out three times for each colour.

Now change the red rose to a beautiful orange chrysanthemum. Breathe this colour in through the soles of your feet and into the sacral chakra, watching it permeate your aura as you exhale.

Next visualize a yellow daffodil and try to feel the vibration of this colour. As you breathe in, bring this clear bright yellow through the soles of your feet and into your solar plexus, breathing it out into your aura.

From the yellow daffodil, change your visualization to a green leaf. Breathe this colour horizontally into your heart chakra and then breathe it out into your aura.

The green leaf then changes into a blue cornflower. Breathe this colour in through the top of your head and into your throat chakra before breathing it out into your aura.

Replace the cornflower with a deep indigo iris. With each inhalation allow this colour to enter through the top of your head and into your brow chakra before exhaling it into your aura.

Lastly, visualize a bunch of tiny violets. Breathe the colour of violet, into your crown chakra and then breathe it out into your aura.

Now relax and try to visualize yourself surrounded by all of these vibrant, dancing colours, each interpenetrating the physical body. When you are ready, breathe in and raise your arms over your head, stretching the whole of your body. Breathe out and bring your arms down to your sides again. Repeat twice more before opening your eyes and sitting up.

COLOUR IN THE CLOTHES WE WEAR

Another way of transmitting colour is through the clothes we wear, which act as a filter through which light passes. Unfortunately, the colour of our clothes is normally dictated by fashion.

If we are wearing a coloured garment for therapeutic purposes, then white must be worn underneath. Failing this, the article of clothing can be worn next to our skin with nothing covering it. If you suffer from high blood pressure, try wearing blue. If, during the winter months, you are sensitive to the cold, wear red, especially on your hands and feet. Didn't our grandparents wear red flannel nightshirts? Just looking at the colour red can help. Try sitting by an electric coal effect fire with just the coal effect alight. I am sure that you will feel warmer even though no heat is being radiated.

As we become more sensitive to colour, we are able to discern which colour or colours we need at any one time. Learning to listen to our bodies enables us to interpret its requirements.

Certain people ascribe individuals to the seasons of the year in terms of colour. They are either a winter, autumn, spring or summer person and they are advised to wear the colours corresponding to these seasons. This is a wonderful way of choosing colours to suit your skin tone but unfortunately its methods cannot be used when working therapeutically with colour.

COLOURS IN FIRST AID

We can use small pieces of cloth as filters which can be placed on any part of the body where there is a problem. Again, only natural fibres should be used. If you are suffering from a sore throat or laryngitis, tie a piece of turquoise silk around your neck, wearing it until the condition improves.

When I was in Florence, helping to run a workshop, I succumbed to a very sore throat and loss of voice. I tied a turquoise silk scarf around my throat and wore it during the day and at night. The following day my throat had considerably improved. I continued the treatment for a further forty-eight hours, by which time my voice had returned and my throat was almost back to normal.

If preferred, small pieces of stained glass can be used as filters (the address where these can be obtained is listed on p. 107). These can be used in two ways – either fitted to a lamp or held over the part of the body to be treated with a light shining through. If it is a sunny day, use the light from the sun.

If you have burnt yourself, use a piece of turquoise glass over the burn, leaving it in position for ten minutes. If you have a small patch of eczema, use yellow stained glass in the same way.

COLOUR IN THE FOOD WE EAT

A very natural way of absorbing colour into our bodies is through the food we eat. I knew a lady who used to prepare 'rainbow meals'. They were delicious and great fun to make. Next time that you are out shopping, take note of the variety of natural coloured foods which are available, and try to select foods which radiate the colour which you feel you might need and include them in your diet.

COLOUR IN THE HOME

Home decoration becomes vitally important the more sensitive we become to colour. To decorate a bedroom, for example, in red or yellow could be disastrous. Red could cause many sleepless nights, while with yellow we could become so detached that we could end up by being well and truly 'spaced out'. The ideal colours are blue or very pale lilac. My hall and therapy room are blue and patients frequently remark how calming and peaceful they find it.

Red is best used in a room where there is a lot of activity, while yellow, the colour associated with the intellect, is good when used in studies or places of intellectual pursuit. Orange, which stands for joy and creativity, can be used in kitchens and children's play rooms. White can be a very isolating and solitary colour, and should therefore always be interspersed with other colours. If you would like more information on the use of colour in decoration, read *Healing Through Colour* by Theo. Gimbel.

ART THERAPY

Another way of using colour therapeutically is through art. Some people can gain inspiration and a sense of well-being simply by looking at beautiful artwork. I found that some of the wonderful artistic creations in Florence were able to lift me into a new dimension of consciousness and health.

To work therapeutically with art, you do not have to be an artist or possess a great gift in this field. It does not matter if you are unable to paint or draw. To work with yourself in this way, you need a set of crayons and a sheet of white or light grey paper. Sit down somewhere quiet and select just three colours from your crayons. Have a chosen piece of music playing in the background and, using your three crayons, interpret, on your sheet of paper, what the music conveys to you. The shapes in the drawing which evolves, should be completely unique to you and should not resemble any known object, such as a flower, house, tree, and so on. Allow your own feelings to be expressed through your hands and on to the paper.

Another way of working in this way is to express disappointment, pain, hurt and anger through your drawing. For this you do not need music, just the three crayons of your choice, and paper. You do not have to create a pretty picture. In fact if you are suffering from any negative emotions, your drawing should be anything but attractive. This does not matter, nobody else is going to see what you have drawn unless you choose to show them, and you are free to destroy it whenever you wish. It is far better to release your feelings in this way then storing them inside yourself where they could, at a later date, manifest as a physical disease. If these methods are worked with under the guidance of a trained art therapist, he/she should be able to interpret your drawings and help you with your problems.

EXPERIENCING COLOUR IN NATURE

Perhaps the most beautiful way to absorb colour is to be like our ancestors and revert back to nature. Endeavouring to spend at least one hour a day in the midst of nature is a wonderful tonic. This can be achieved by sitting or working in the garden, walking through parks, or in the countryside – a pursuit which should be done throughout all the seasons of the year. Each season brings its own range of colours and with them come very special healing powers. Whenever possible, I sit in my garden to work. To me, the inspirational and healing power with which I am surrounded is truly awe inspiring.

If you are interested in experiencing the healing power of colour, may I suggest, that you start your journey by walking every day in nature's healing environment.

7

Taking It Further

I F YOU HAVE found the information given in this book
interesting, you may feel that you would like to expand
your knowledge on the subject; experience colour therapy for
yourself; train to become a colour practitioner; or learn more
about colour in order that you may use it in conjunction with
any other therapy that you are practising. Alternatively, you
might like to learn how to use colour in decoration, in dress,
or in art. We are affected by colour, however we may use it.

There are many excellent books on the market which
explore every aspect of colour, and some of these are listed
at the end of this chapter. If you belong to a local library,
check to see if they have any of the books that you wish to
read before going out and buying them. If they do not have
them, they will often order them for you. On the other hand,
you may wish to buy them for future reference, especially if
you intend to take your interest in colour further.

Should you decide that you would like to be treated with
colour and do not know of anyone practising in your area, there
are several ways of finding your nearest colour practitioner.
The first is by contacting The Institute for Complementary
Medicine (ICM). The ICM is a registered charity with three
main areas of work: 1. information service to the general
public; 2. recognition of training standards of practitioners;
and 3. encouragement of research.

The ICM will either give you the names and addresses of
practitioners living in or around your area, or they will
give you the name and telephone number of one of the

accepted training schools. In the case of the latter, ring the school and ask if they can give you the name of a qualified colour practitioner in your area. Most schools have a register of the practitioners who have qualified through them and will send out copies to enquirers. It is important that whoever treats you should be qualified. To find out, ask them where they trained and then telephone the school to find out if they are on the register. It is important to do this if the person treating you comes either through recommendation or an advertisement for at present it is very easy for anybody to set up as a practitioner in many branches of complementary medicine. Fortunately, as British standards are being brought into line with other countries, this will become much more difficult in the near future. Treatment given by unqualified people can be dangerous, can damage the therapy by giving it a bad name, and can undermine those who have studied hard in order to practise it.

Another association which gives information on colour therapy and colour practitioners is 'The International Association for Colour Therapists' (IACT). This is affiliated to the Institute for Complementary Medicine, and was started by Theo. Gimbel in 1984 to promote colour consciousness in all forms of healing and complementary therapies. Its aims and objectives are:

1. To establish colour healing as a significant branch of complementary therapy.
2. To determine professional standards of practice in the use of colour therapy.
3. To improve the understanding and use of colour in healing, health, beauty, fashion, décor, industry and complementary therapies.
4. To make it easier for people to find out more about colour and how to avail themselves of colour therapy.

The associate membership is open to anyone who is interested in or working with colour in any field and to anyone who is studying colour at a recognized school. To obtain full membership, graduation from a recognized school is required plus a minimum of three years' professional experience in the therapeutic use of colour.

The activities of IACT include making information about training in the use of colour available through lectures, courses, workships, seminars and conferences; helping and supporting members and providing opportunities for them to contact others who are interested in or working with colour; promoting periodic publications throughout the year; making colour therapy available to the public; and keeping members informed about research in the use of colour.

Should you wish to train as a colour practitioner, there are several schools which run training courses. I would advise that before embarking upon a lengthy and sometimes costly course, you check that the qualifications offered by the school of your choice have been accepted by the ICM as reaching the required standard. The duration and cost of training differs from school to school, and it is advantageous to glean information from several schools before making a choice.

To give some idea of what is expected of a student and what training involves, I will cite the two schools with which I have had personal contact.

The first is The Maitreya School of Healing which was founded in 1974 by Lily Cornford and Ronald Leech (known to most people as Joseph). For many years, Lily and Joseph worked with small groups of people, teaching the information which was transmitted through their intuition from a higher level of consciousness. Over the years, more and more people were attracted to their work, and by 1990 their work had grown to such proportions that it moved to its present address (see List of Addresses on p. 106).

The philosophy of the Maitreya School taken from their curriculum is:

> We aspire to prepare healers for the healing work of the Aquarian age by transmitting knowledge, cultivating Heart, instilling responsibility. The school hopes to provide an environment in which the healer can purify his/her own vehicle of manifestation; discover what service she/he can offer to the kingdoms of nature (human, animal, plant and mineral kingdom) and become sensitive to the presence and healing qualities of the angels and fairies.

Training to become a practitioner through the Maitreya School consists of thirteen weekly training sessions. At the end of this period, the students are given both a practical and theoretical examination. If they are successful in passing these, they are then expected to undertake one hundred hours of training at the school under the supervision of a qualified practitioner.

The Maitreya School also runs a Mental Colour Therapy Clinic which provides treatment by qualified mental colour practitioners. The charge for adults is minimal and treatment is free of charge for children up to school-leaving age. The Maitreya School believes that the children's treatment becomes the school's investment towards creating a more spiritual future for the planet.

The second school with which I have had personal contact and where I have taught is the Hygeia College of Colour Therapy, founded by Theo. Gimbel in 1976. Over many years, Theo. has developed a comprehensive system for the therapeutic use of colour energies, and his work acknowledges that of earlier researchers such as J.W. Goethe, Rudolf Steiner, Edwin Babbitt and Dinshah P. Ghadiali. The College believes and teaches the principle that colour works at the subtle level of the auric body and with its related chakras. The physical disturbances are prefigured by imbalances in the aura which the energies of colour are able to harmonize. In so doing, negative patterns are released from the body, and this allows natural healing to take place. Attention is directed at replacing negative thoughts and emotions with positive life-affirming ones. The ultimate goals of therapy are peace and joy, and these are worked towards with insight, discipline and spiritual inspiration.

The training given for a colour practitioner at Hygeia College takes approximately two years. It consists of six weekend foundation courses, a two-week residential course, and a probationary year.

The six weekend foundation courses cover colour, healing, music, form, counselling, and colour and its application to health. After each of these weekends, the students are asked to write an essay on their understanding of the weekend. At the end of the six foundation courses, they are expected to write a dissertation of not less than 7,000 words before attending the advanced course. Their dissertation can be on any aspect of colour about which they feel drawn to write. The six weekend courses can be taken residentially at Hygeia College or non-residentially in London.

The two-week advanced course, which is residential and held at Hygeia College, incorporates three examination papers (two on colour therapy and one on anatomy and physiology); practical tests; interviews; and lectures given by practitioners from different complementary disciplines.

If and when students have reached the required standard, they are expected to work with friends and relatives for a year, submitting twelve case histories to the college. At the end of the year, if all is satisfactory, their name is added to the Hygeia Register of Colour Practitioners.

After qualifying, should a student wish to teach colour therapy, they have to study for their diploma. This normally takes a further two years.

For those of you who would like some insight into colour therapy before embarking upon a training course, and for those who would just like to know something about colour therapy, introductory days are run in London.

Other schools which teach colour from basic to diploma level are 'Aura Soma' and 'Know Yourself Through Colour'. The addresses and telephone numbers of these schools are given in the List of Addresses.

There are also schools which include colour and healing in their syllabus, and these may be of interest to those who do not wish to embark upon a full training course. Three such schools are: Living Art run by Jane Cory Wright MIACT; Promethus run by Dr Carol Brierley MIACT; and Living a Rainbow run by Noelle Lever MIACT. Their addresses and telephone numbers can be obtained from IACT.

Weekend courses on the use of colour in conjunction with reflexology are run in London. These are aimed at qualified reflexologists who wish to use colour with their treatment. During the course of these weekends, participants explore colour and its meaning, and the aura and the chakras (where these are located on the spinal reflex of the feet and the importance of working with them). Techniques are shown to help students become more sensitive to the vibrational frequencies of colour, thereby enabling a greater understanding of the effect that colour has on each individual. The group is then taught how the Reflexology Crystal Torch can be used in conjunction with a normal reflexology treatment to apply colour to the reflexes of the feet in order to promote healing. For details of these workshops, contact the author.

Courses are also run for those who wish to work with colour and yoga. These courses are suitable for people who are complete beginners as well as for those who have some knowledge of either yoga or colour. Again details can be obtained from the author.

Having read this book, should you decide to work with colour in any of its many facets, I wish you the joy and wonder that it has afforded me.

May the light from the Eternal Source which radiates from your heart and is expressed in the living dancing colours which surround you, bless you with health, harmony and joy.

Addresses

The Institute for Complementary Medicine
Unit 5, Tavern Quay
Commercial Centre
Rope Street
London SE16 1TX
Tel: 0171 237 5165

The International Association for Colour Therapy
137 Hendon Lane
Finchley
London N3

The Hygeia College of Colour Therapy
Brook House
Avening
Tetbury
Gloucestershire GL8 8NS
Tel: 01453 832150
London Contact: Pauline Wills 0181 204 7672

Aura Soma
South Road
Tetford
Horncastle
Lincolnshire LN9 6QL
Tel: 01507 533441

Addresses

Know Yourself Through Colour
Marie Louise Lacy
3a Bath Road
Worthing
Sussex
BN11 3NU
Tel: 01903 216311

Pauline Wills
9 Wyndale Avenue
Kingsbury
London NW9 9PT
Tel: 0181 204 7672

Resources

Full Length Silks
Colour Crystal Torch
Water Solarizer
Colour Therapy Instrument
Colour Space Illuminator
Stained Glass Filters

All obtainable from Hygeia Studios

Colour Reflexology Torch
Obtainable from Pauline Wills

Further Reading

Alpen, F. *Exploring Atlantis*, Arizona Metaphysical Society, 1981.

Anderson, M. *Colour Healing*, The Aquarian Press, 1979.

Ghadiali, D. *Spectro-Chrome Metry Encyclopedia*, Spectro-Chrome Institute, 1939.

Gimbel, T. *Form, Sound, Colour & Healing*, C.W. Daniel 1987.

——*Healing Through Colour*, C.W. Daniel, 1980.

Goethe, J.W. *The Theory of Colour*.

Hunt, R. *The Seven Keys to Colour Healing*, C.W. Daniel, 1968.

Huxley, A. *The Doors of Perception*, Chatto & Windus, 1968.

——*Moksha*, Penguin Books, 1977.

Iyengar, B.K.S. *Body the Shrine, Yoga the Light*, B.I. Taraporewala, Bombay, 1978.

Karagulla, S. and Van Gelder Kunz, D. *The Chakras and the Human Energy Field*, Theosophical Publishing House, 1989.

Lacy, M.L. *Know Yourself Through Colour*, Aquarian Press, 1989.

Liberman, J. *Light, Medicine of the Future*, Bear and Co, 1991.

Lynes, B. *The Healing of Cancer*, Marcus Books, Canada, 1989.

Mascero. J. (ed.) *The Upanishads*, Penguin Classic.

Ouseley, S.G. *The Power of the Rays*, L.N. Fowler & Co Ltd, 1961.

Brooke Simpkins, E. *New Light on the Eyes*, Vincent Stuart, 1958.

Wall, V. *The Miracle of Colour Healing*, Aquarian Press, 1990.

Wills, P. *The Reflexology and Colour Workbook*, Element Books, 1992.

Wills, P. and Gimbel, T. *16 Steps to Health and Energy*, Foulsham, 1992.

New Larousse Encyclopedia of Mythology (Introduction by Robert Graves) Hamlyn, 1959.

Index

visualization 8, 54, 70, 81,
  85, 86, 87, 88, 89, 90,
  91, 92, 94, 96
vocal chords 54

Wall, Vicky 68
Wehr, Dr Thomas 13
white 2, 3, 9, 31, 34,
  36, 63, 67

wrist 74

X-rays 10

yellow 1, 3, 4, 9, 18, 19,
  29, 32, 33, 34, 36, 50,
  63, 84, 88, 95

yoga 6, 43, 53, 69–70,
  85–93

Zeus 28, 30, 31